DIGNITY, FREEDOM, AND GRACE

D1599281

DIGNITY, FREEDOM, AND GRACE

Christian Perspectives on HIV, AIDS, and Human Rights

Edited by Gillian Paterson and Callie Long

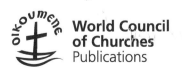

World Council of Churches Publications

DIGNITY, FREEDOM, AND GRACE:
Christian Perspectives on HIV, AIDS, and Human Rights
Edited by Gillian Paterson and Callie Long

WCC Publications is the book publishing programme of the World Council of Churches. Founded in 1948, the WCC promotes Christian unity in faith, witness and service for a just and peaceful world. A global fellowship, the WCC brings together 345 Protestant, Orthodox, Anglican and other churches representing more than 550 million Christians in 110 countries and works cooperatively with the Roman Catholic Church.

Opinions expressed in WCC Publications are those of the authors.

The Ecumenical Advocacy Alliance, an ecumenical initiative of the World Council of Churches, is a global network of churches and related organizations committed to campaigning together on common concerns for justice and human dignity. Current campaign issues are HIV and AIDS, food security, and sustainable agriculture. The EAA gratefully acknowledges the support of the Norwegian Agency for Development Cooperation (Norad) and UNAIDS.

Cover design, book design and typesetting: Michelle Cook / 4 Seasons Book Design
Cover image: Jedrzej Chelminski/EAA
ISBN: 978-2-8254-1679-2

World Council of Churches
150 route de Ferney, P.O. Box 2100
1211 Geneva 2, Switzerland
http://publications.oikoumene.org

Contents

Preface   ix

Contributors   xiii

Abbreviations   xix

Prologue: Human Rights: Nothing to Be Afraid of   xxi
    Gillian Paterson

Part One: Critical Issues   1

1. What's Wrong with Rights?   3
    Julie Clague

2. Part of the Solution and Part of the Problem?   12
    Sally Smith

3. Why Stigma Matters   22
    Suzette Moses-Burton

4. Sexual and Reproductive Health Rights for Young Women   28
    Hendrica Okondo

5. Health Care, HIV, and Human Rights: An Approach That Works   34
    Callie Long

Part Two: Contextual Struggles   43

6. Reflecting on the Role of Networks of People Living with HIV   45
    JP Mokgethi-Heath and Phumzile Mabizela

7. Evidence and Experience of Key Populations   49
    Sex Work, Human Rights and the Church   49
    Peninah Mwangi

My Role as an Advocate for the International Network of People Who Use Drugs (INPUD) 51
  Mags Maher
Sexuality and Self-Worth 55
  "Marcus"
8. Just Care and the Image of God: An Orthodox Perspective on HIV, AIDS, and Human Rights 58
  Geevarghese Coorilos
9. Theological Challenges and Opportunities in Addressing Human Rights, Sexuality, and HIV: An African Perspective 60
  Ezra Chitando
10. From Apartheid Activism to AIDS Advocacy: A South African Perspective 66
  Callie Long
11. "Let Grace Be Total": The Ministry of the United Church of Christ in the Philippines 73
  Erlinda N. Senturias
12. Stigma, HIV, and Diverse Sexuality: Examples of Faith Responses Affirming Human Dignity 75
  JP Mokgethi-Heath
13. A Common Language for Human Rights, Faith, and HIV: An Example of Ministry in the Philippines 80
  Richard R. Mickley
14. As Science Advances . . . the Human Heart Hardens: A Brazilian Perspective 85
  Ester Lisboa
15. The Armenian Apostolic Church: An Orthodox Church's Response to the Challenges of HIV and AIDS 89
  Karine Kocharian
16. Living by Faith in Challenging Times: A Caribbean View on What It Means to Say, "God Will Take Care of Us" 95
  Garth Minott

Part Three: Some Theological Entry Points 101

17. The Redemption of God's Good Gift of Sexuality 102
   Michael Schuenemeyer

18. The Image of God: Recognizing God within Key Populations
   Ijeoma Ajibade 109

19. Gender Inequality and Human Rights:
   A Prophetic Trinitarian Anthropology 116
   Nontando Hadebe

Epilogue: Dignity, Freedom, and Grace 123
   Gillian Paterson

Notes 126
Resources 132

Preface

"By 2020, 90% of all people living with HIV will know their HIV status. By 2020, 90% of all people with diagnosed HIV infection will receive sustained antiretroviral therapy. By 2020, 90% of all people receiving antiretroviral therapy will have viral suppression."

– UNAIDS Target of "90-90-90"

The aim of this book is to provide background, context, and theological "tools" to support individuals and faith communities seeking to explore the role of human rights in their responses to HIV.

Engaging with this epidemic has been a learning experience, especially for faith communities. In particular, it is now widely accepted that biomedical approaches to epidemics alone are inadequate. This is particularly true when social and structural inequalities increase vulnerability to HIV infection, when people living with HIV or AIDS face stigmatization and discrimination, and when groups or individuals who are particularly vulnerable to HIV are ostracized or treated as criminals. Communities of faith play important roles in setting and changing social norms and influencing public policy and legislation. This influence has played out in both positive and negative ways in the response to HIV.

At the global level, the HIV response is articulated within a framework of human rights. There is increasing consensus that for progress to be made toward targets like 90-90-90, or toward the ultimate goal of zero new infections and zero AIDS-related deaths, it is necessary for responses to HIV and AIDS to be clearly rooted in a human rights approach. This framing has exposed sharp differences and sparked, on occasion, confrontation and condemnation from all sides. At times, this has been accompanied by a refusal to dialogue, listen, or seek to understand.

Now, more than ever, with the urgency to scale up HIV testing and linkage to care, there is no single approach that will achieve the targets alone. It will take collaboration across all the sectors and the active engagement of social and religious actors to address not only the biomedical challenges, but also the socio-cultural and structural challenges that increase vulnerability and block progress.

Beginning in 2011, therefore, the Ecumenical Advocacy Alliance (EAA) has been seeking to address increasing polarization of positions through a series of face-to-face international consultations. An ecumenical initiative of the World Council of Churches, the EAA is a global network of churches and related organizations committed to campaigning together on common concerns for justice and human dignity. These consultations have recognized sensitivities on all sides but also pointed to common ground between the human rights framework and theological concepts of justice and human dignity, shared commitments, and the need to foster open dialogue at local and national levels. The present volume is one outcome of that process.

Addressing emotive and potentially divisive topics in a sensitive way through dialogue is a difficult task in itself, and the development of this publication has been more like a journey than a writing assignment with a pre-determined end. A major challenge has been that while EAA's campaign on HIV has a strong foundation in upholding and protecting human rights, we recognize that within EAA's participating organizations there are different attitudes, language, approaches, and responses based on theology, history, and context.

In this publication, we have brought together a wide variety of perspectives. These can only reflect in part the full range of positions and issues raised by the nexus of human rights, HIV, and faith. What has united all of the contributors and input from the meetings is the common belief in a loving, creator God, and the compassionate Christ, ever standing in solidarity with those made vulnerable and marginalized from communities. However, do not expect that our authors will agree with each other, or that you will agree with all of them. The articles and essays in this publication reflect the particular experience and perspectives of the writers themselves. Some may inspire you, some may make you uncomfortable, and some could make you angry. We hope, in fact, that at least some of this happens. Our aim here is to raise the key issues, promote honest, respectful discussion, and help to bring people together in the ongoing search for resources to assist dialogue and action.

On behalf of the Ecumenical Advocacy Alliance, I wish to express our great appreciation to those who have made this book possible:

Gillian Paterson and Callie Long, who accepted the invitation to co-edit the publication in its concept stage, and whose skills, experience, knowledge, and patience have shaped all the creative, diverse input into a sensible and inspiring whole;

Our expert editorial committee – Ezra Chitando, Julie Clague, Nontando Hadebe, J. P. Mokgethi-Heath, and Sally Smith – which helped to guide the initial framework and process for the publication, contributed key articles, and provided wise and invaluable advice throughout the process;

Lyn van Rooyen, who agreed to our request to organize the resources section before the size of the task became apparent, and who, through her expertise and experience, has honed the lists at the back of this book into a usable format;

The many participants in EAA's consultations on human rights, HIV, and faith, with special thanks for their willingness to bring their experiences of pain, conviction, compassion, and dignity to the task of sharpening a common vision of what is needed in order to overcome HIV-related stigma and discrimination;

The participants of the October 2014 colloquium, whose incredible inspiration and insight have turned the idea of a publication into a living reality and whose rich contributions could have filled several more books;

Former EAA staff who have shepherded this process over many years, particularly Peter Prove, Ruth Foley, and Anne-Laure Jan;

Those organizations that have made the publication possible through their financial contributions: UNAIDS and the Norwegian Agency for Development Cooperation (Norad) through the "EAA, World YWCA and WCC-EHAIA Consortium";

And finally, to you, the reader, for being willing to enter the dialogue.

—*Sara Speicher*
World Council of Churches – Ecumenical Advocacy Alliance

Contributors

REV. IJEOMA AJIBADE is a Church of England priest, ministering in a London parish and at Southwark Cathedral in London. Alongside her ministry, she has worked in the UK public sector for 27 years, including trying to mobilize the church to address HIV through its ministry and mission. She has developed training courses on HIV for clergy in the diocese of Southwark, and helped set up the Kaleidoscope Trust, an organization working for the human rights of lesbian and gay people in countries where it is a crime to be gay.

EZRA CHITANDO is the anglophone Theology Consultant to the WCC programme on Ecumenical HIV and AIDS Initiatives and Advocacy (EHAIA), and he is Associate Professor of History and Phenomenology of Religion at the University of Zimbabwe. He has published extensively on religion in Africa, sexuality, and health. Among his recent publications is *In the Name of Jesus! Healing in the Age of HIV* (2013, WCC Publications).

JULIE CLAGUE teaches Christian theology and ethics at the University of Glasgow, UK. She is co-chair of the HIV and Maternal Health Learning Hub for the Joint Learning Initiative on Faith and Local Communities (www.jliflc. com), and a member of CAFOD's HIV Advisory Group. She co-edits the journal *Political Theology* (www.politicaltheology.com)

METROPOLITAN DR GEEVARGHESE COORILOS is a bishop of the Syrian Orthodox Church and the Metropolitan of Niranam. He is currently serving as Moderator of the Commission on World Mission and Evangelism of the World Council of Churches.

DR NONTANDO HADEBE lectures in theology at St Augustine College South Africa. Key research interests include gender, HIV and AIDS, feminist/womanist theologies, and Trinitarian theology. She presents radio programs and is a member of the Circle of Concerned African Women Theologians.

KARINE KOCHARIAN is Program Coordinator for the World Council of Churches Armenia Round Table Foundation, focused on HIV, AIDS and family wellness: a post she has held since 2012. She received her first degree in psychology from Gyumri Pedagogical Institute, Armenia, and her Master's Degree in Public Administration from Grand Valley State University, Michigan, USA.

ESTER LISBOA is programme staff of KOINONIA Ecumenical Presence and Service in Brazil. She is a social worker by profession and commissioned representative of the National Council of Christian Churches of Brazil (CONIC – Conselho Nacional de Igrejas Cristãs do Brasil) at CNAIDS (STD, AIDS, and Viral Hepatitis National Committee, Brazil).

CALLIE LONG is a media development practitioner, journalist, and organizational communicator with a specialized focus on conflict, health and AIDS advocacy. She is working on her Ph.D. in the Humanities at Brock University in Canada, researching HIV-related stigma within a trauma theory framework.

REV. PHUMZILE MABIZELA is the Executive Director of the International Network of Religious Leaders Living with or Personally Affected by HIV and AIDS (INERELA+). Rev. Mabizela is also a member of the Circle of Concerned African Women Theologians. Before joining INERELA+ she was employed by Norwegian Church Aid as the Senior Policy Advisor on Gender Justice in Southern Africa and served as the Chief Executive Officer of the KwaZulu-Natal Christian Council. Rev. Mabizela is a passionate gender, HIV and AIDS activist.

MAGS MAHER is a drug and alcohol specialist/consultant in the UK and an advocate for the International Network of People Who Use Drugs (INPUD). She is currently area coordinator for EuroNPUD.

MARCUS is a young man from the Philippines, whose name has been changed to protect his identity.

BISHOP RICHARD R. MICKLEY was born in Ohio, USA, and has been a missionary in the Philippines for 24 years. In the early 1980s, as a Metropolitan Community Church pastor in Los Angeles, he cared for gay men dying of a then-mysterious disease. While serving as MCC pastor in Auckland, New Zealand, he was Coordinator of the Interfaith AIDS Ministry Network sponsored by the National Council of Churches, and in Manila, he was Coordinator of the Faith-based AIDS Ministry of the AIDS Society of the Philippines. In 2011 he was appointed as Bishop of the Catholic Diocese of One Spirit Philippines, and founded the Well Wellness Method for holistic well-being of people living with HIV.

REV. FR GARTH MINOTT teaches Introduction to Ministry, Christian Ethics, Introduction to Psychology, Introduction to Theology, Pastoral Counselling and Christian Worship at United Theological College of the West Indies, where he has served as Deputy President for a two-year term. He is currently undertaking Ph.D. studies, focusing on Christian Ethics, Social Justice, and HIV and AIDS in the Caribbean. Fr Minott received the CIBC RBC Bank Unsung Hero award for his work in the area of HIV and AIDS and was acclaimed as a trailblazer in the field of social justice advocacy for HIV.

REV. JP MOKGETHI-HEATH is an Anglican Priest from Southern Africa, now working for the Church of Sweden. His personal experience as a religious leader living with HIV led him to co-found INERELA+ (International Network of Religious Leaders Living with or Personally Affected by HIV). While currently working as Policy Advisor on HIV and Theology for the Church of Sweden, he continues to serve on boards and reference groups on HIV for the World Council of Churches and the United Nations.

SUZETTE MOSES-BURTON served as Executive Director of the Global Network of People Living with HIV (GNP+) from January 2014 to January 2016, and has been an advocate and leader for people living with HIV for over 20 years. Formerly the HIV/AIDS Programme Manager for St Maarten, she chaired the Caribbean Regional Network of Persons living with HIV/AIDS and sat as a board member of the St Maarten AIDS Foundation, the Caribbean Coalition of National AIDS Programme Coordinators, and the Pan Caribbean Partnership against HIV.

PENINAH MWANGI is executive director of the Bar Hostess Empowerment & Support Programme (BHESP) and is chairperson of the African Sexworkers Alliance (ASWA). BHESP is an organization for and by sex workers, women having sex with women, women using drugs and bar hostesses in Kenya to advocate for their rights and recognition. ASWA is a sex work movement/ network formed in 2009 by empowered sex worker leaders, women's activists and NGOs who support the rights of sex workers and publically denounce the stigma, discrimination, and criminalization of sex work.

HENDRICA OKONDO joined World YWCA in 2010 as the Global Programme Manager, Sexual and Reproductive Health and Rights and HIV and AIDS. She has worked in public health in Kenya, and has also served as Gender Adviser at the UN World Food Programme, Programme Manager for UNIFEM South Sudan, and Country Programme Manager for UNIFEM Tanzania. For over 20 years she has advocated for implementation of key global commitments on rights for women, young women, and girls.

DR GILLIAN PATERSON is co-editor of this book. She is a research fellow and visiting lecturer at Heythrop College, University of London, and co-ordinates the Catholic Network for Population and Development. She has worked in the field of HIV and AIDS since the mid-1990s, often with the Ecumenical Advocacy Alliance and World Council of Churches. She is the author of books and articles on faith and health, especially in relation to HIV.

REV. MICHAEL SCHUENEMEYER is Executive Director of the United Church of Christ AIDS Network in the USA, where he is also an Executive in the Office for Health and Wholeness Advocacy within the Church's Justice and Witness Ministries and Wider Church Ministries.

DR ERLINDA N. SENTURIAS is a physician, educator, ecumenical activist, and former staff member of the World Council of Churches. In 2014, she was appointed to the Philippines' new Human Rights Victims Claims Board.

SALLY SMITH is senior adviser for faith-based organizations in UNAIDS. Having worked for UNAIDS for ten years in Community Mobilization and Partnerships, she now has overall responsibility for UNAIDS liaison with faith-based organizations (FBOs) and religions. She is also doing a doctorate at Glasgow University, UK. She has over 30 years' experience working with

FBOs and civil society engaged in sexual and reproductive health and rights and AIDS, including with networks of people living with HIV and FBOs from the Buddhist, Christian, Hindu, and Islamic traditions

SARA SPEICHER has worked with the Ecumenical Advocacy Alliance since 2004 as communications consultant and served as EAA interim executive director from May 2014 – February 2015. She previously served as communication officer and director of public information for the World Council of Churches (WCC), and continues to provide communication services to the WCC-EAA, the World Association for Christian Communication, and others.

LYN VAN ROOYEN is director of CABSA (the Christian AIDS Bureau of Southern Africa). She is passionate about the role of faith communities in a competent HIV response. She has been involved in the NGO sector since 2004 and serves on various NGO boards. She holds a BCur (Nursing) (RAU) and an MBA (University of Wales).

Abbreviations

AIDS	acquired immune deficiency syndrome
BHESP	Bar Hostess Empowerment & Support Programme
CAFOD	Catholic Fund for Overseas Development
CEDAW	Convention on the Elimination of all Forms of Discrimination against Women
CONIC	National Council of Christian Churches of Brazil
EAA	Ecumenical Advocacy Alliance
EHAIA	Ecumenical HIV and AIDS Initiatives and Advocacy (formerly Ecumenical HIV/AIDS Initiative in Africa)
FBOs	faith-based organizations
GIN-SSOGIE	Global Interfaith Network for People of all Sexes, Sexual Orientations, Gender Identities and Expressions
GNP+	Global Network of People Living with HIV
HIV	human immunodeficiency virus
HPV	human papilloma virus
ICAAP	International Congress on AIDS in Asia and the Pacific
ILGA	International Lesbian and Gay Association
INERELA+	International network of religious leaders living with or personally affected by HIV or AIDS
INPUD	International Network of People Who Use Drugs

LGBTI	lesbian, gay, bisexual, transgender, and intersex
MSM	men who have sex with men
NGO	non-governmental organization
PLHIV	People living with HIV
SRHR	sexual and reproductive health and rights
SSDDIM	stigma, shame, denial, discrimination, inaction, mis-action
STD	sexually transmitted disease
UCCP	United Church of Christ in the Philippines
UDHR	Universal Declaration of Human Rights
UN	United Nations
UNAIDS	Joint United Nations Programme on HIV/AIDS
UNFPA	United Nations Population Fund
WCC	World Council of Churches
YWCA	Young Women's Christian Association

"Key populations" is often used to refer to both vulnerable and most-at-risk populations. These include people living with HIV, men who have sex with men, transgender people, people who inject drugs, and sex workers. This also includes groups who are particularly vulnerable to HIV infection in certain situations or contexts, such as adolescents (particularly adolescent girls), orphans, street children, people in closed settings (such as prisons), people with disabilities, and migrant and mobile workers.

Human Rights: Nothing to Be Afraid Of

Gillian Paterson

"We have created a false dichotomy between faith and human rights. The human rights discourse began with 'in His image He created them.' No human being stands outside this image."

– Participant in the October 2014 colloquium

Why this book?

The idea of human rights is perhaps the most influential philosophical and political idea of our time. "Rights," understood as attributes that every human being possesses simply by virtue of being human, have become the foundation stone of much international discourse.

Christians, in recent history, have a fine record in championing this idea. For example, the World Council of Churches (WCC) was involved in the drafting of the original United Nations Declaration of Human Rights, while John Paul II insisted on their crucial place in the struggle for freedom. In the process, the concept of rights, which started out as a philosophical basis for political organization and change, has become a part of Christian moral discourse: for many Christians, a fundamental ingredient of God's moral purposes. Today, indeed, human rights principles may claim for themselves a quasi-religious universality that in turn can seem to take precedence over all other claims to truth. In Chapter 1 (*What's Wrong with Rights?*) Julie Clague gives an account how this came to be.

However, this understanding of human rights is neither unanimously nor universally endorsed. By some people, Christians and otherwise, the human rights agenda is viewed as a tool of secular Western imperialism, designed to be a vehicle for Western consumerism and materialism, to undermine faith and to destabilize local cultural values and structures of authority. For example, promoting rights for women and girls, which is a fundamental principle of UN thinking, may be interpreted as an attack on local cultures, authority structures, and in particular on the integrity of the traditional family. Religious belief is sometimes used as an argument for denying human rights to some groups of individuals. For example, in the name of religion gay men have been persecuted, imprisoned, or murdered, and "key populations" are excluded from community. Appeals for access by sex workers to sexual and reproductive health (SRH) advice, or by drug injectors to harm-reduction facilities, have been resisted as tools of morally bankrupt Western liberalism intent on colonizing the rest of the world with its sinful beliefs. Even in societies where there is, at community level, a strong sense of mutual responsibility and commitment, the idea that individual rights should ever take precedence over community rights has sometimes been interpreted as a manifestation of an alien individualism.

It must equally be admitted that the language of rights has become, to some extent, debased, as for example when it is used (as it often is) to advocate for entitlements that involve disregarding the needs of others and the basic demands of justice: what Julie Clague, in her essay, describes as "an epidemic of rightsism." It is interesting that Pope Francis, whose commitment to the poor and downtrodden is not in question, has been cautious in his use of the language of rights, taking more interest in structural problems that talk of individual rights cannot solve, and may indeed make worse. Human rights, by his interpretation, are to be used less for promoting human freedom or the concerns of individuals than for achieving social justice. He said, in 2013: "Sadly, even human rights can be used as a justification of the inordinate defense of individual rights or the rights of the richer peoples. . . . To speak properly of our own rights, we need to broaden our perspective and to hear the cry of other peoples and other regions than our own country."[1]

In 2011, with the support and participation of UN agencies, the Ecumenical Advocacy Alliance (EAA) and its global partners initiated an international process of reflection designed to explore faith perspectives on HIV, AIDS, and human rights. Bringing together people living with, working with, researching on, or personally affected by HIV or AIDS, EAA invited them to share and record their own thoughts and experiences. These conversations were always lively, sometimes uncomfortable, and often deeply moving. Nevertheless, they provided confirmation of the view that there is indeed a problem.

The present publication is one outcome of this process. Written out of a particular faith tradition (Christianity), it makes no claim to be representative of other faiths, although many of the issues it addresses are encountered in similar ways within other faith traditions. Its starting point lies in the realities of the lived experience of people who are, themselves, subject to the human rights abuses we are seeking to address. It has brought together a team of writers, all living with, personally affected by, or working in the field of HIV and AIDS, most of them Christian, in the hope that their stories will be a resource and a source of encouragement to organizations, groups, and individuals working in both fields.

What to expect

Part One explores some overarching issues, starting with Julie Clague's careful account (already mentioned) of the development of modern human rights thinking. In Chapter 2, Sally Smith speaks from her position as Senior Advisor on Religion at UNAIDS, giving a powerful personal account of her experience of "standing in the gap," brokering conversations between two sets of values. On the one hand, she says, there is the discourse of faith, with its own set of values and beliefs; on the other, there is the discourse of human rights and of sexual and reproductive health. One of the fault-lines exposed by the HIV epidemic, she suggests, has been the distrust and fear that exists between these two discourses and the cultures and beliefs they support.

Meanwhile, abuses of human rights have severely undermined the capacity of societies to respond to HIV and AIDS. She cites the neglect and stigmatization of orphans, the refusal to provide realistic, truthful education, or gender rules that deny to women the right to say "no" to sex encounters or to influence decisions on family size. Often, she says, this is reinforced by moral teaching that assumes an ideal of family and community life that does not, in fact, exist, which may be accompanied by a communal silence on the subject of abuses, even when it is common knowledge that they are taking place.

Most of our writers have stressed the toxic effects of HIV-related stigma, joining their voices to those who already urge faith groups to review their own teachings and practices. Chapter 3, in particular, is a moving personal account of one woman's personal and professional encounters with stigma, written by Suzette Moses-Burton, former executive director of GNP+ (the Global Network of People living with HIV or AIDS). Then in Chapter 4, Hendrica Okondo discusses the particular vulnerability of young women and girls, and describes how her own organization, the World YWCA, has made a difference.

In Chapter 5, "Health Care, HIV and Human Rights: An Approach That Works," my co-editor, Callie Long, argues that religion, though it may be part of the problem, is also part of the solution. Some of the earliest responses to the epidemic came from faith-based organizations active in health care. Christian churches, in particular, have an honourable history in this respect. But they have also, sometimes, been responsible for stigma-driven attitudes that failed to acknowledge the reality of vulnerability based on gender or sexual orientation. When healthcare providers (or others) encourage people to view HIV as a moral issue rather than a virus, it undermines public health initiatives and discourages people from being tested, seeking treatment, or changing behaviour.

Within the formal healthcare agenda, too, there are conflicting approaches to rights, with many international policy-makers arguing that a traditional public health approach (which is to do with protecting the population at large through compulsory testing and notification of contacts) should outweigh a strictly medical one (where the primary duty is toward the individual patient and the principles of confidentiality that come with that commitment). In justifying this latter approach, the notion of "AIDS-exceptionalism" has been widely (though not universally) promoted to urge a degree of exemption, for HIV and AIDS, from routine approaches to communicable infection.

It must be stressed that the present publication is not attempting to take a particular position on these arguments, but simply to point out their impact on the issues we are addressing: namely Christian perspectives on HIV, AIDS, and human rights. For it often turns out that effective HIV control ends up by offending both the above groups within the medical establishment, and also many religiously motivated groups. For example, condoms and clean syringes are important elements in prevention strategies, even if many people oppose them; and the tracing of sexual partners is a significant part of public health strategy, even if human rights advocates resist it.

Again, the concept of the "key populations" is commonly used to refer to groups of individuals who are particularly vulnerable to infection, and good public health practice suggests they should be particularly encouraged to seek help. When sex workers, injecting drug users, and men who have sex with men are stigmatized or treated as criminals, it is likely to have the reverse effect.

Part Two of this book, therefore, consists of a series of moving accounts, some of them highly personal, which speak to us of the contextual struggles individuals and communities of faith have taken on in responding to HIV. We open with the experience of individuals from Africa, Asia, and Europe who are themselves living with or particularly vulnerable to HIV or AIDS, and with those regional and international organizations which embody that experience. We have two very different Orthodox perspectives: first, from India, a discussion of the notion of Just Care; then an account, from Armenia, of a service for people living with HIV, their families, and their survivors, which embodies the best principles of human rights without ever using the phrase itself. We hear from African contexts about how the epidemic is influenced by its political context in post-apartheid South Africa as well as in the wider context of post-colonial Africa.

Also emphasizing the importance of political and intellectual context, we hear from the Philippines, from Brazil, and from the Caribbean. An Anglican priest speaks of the struggle to keep faith in a sometimes-hostile social and ecclesial situation, and a Namibian living in Sweden of the particularly acute challenges faced by people with diverse sexualities. We are deeply grateful to this remarkable group of people for sharing their thoughts and experience so honestly with us.

For Part Three, we asked three Christian theologians to explore some of the contributions that Christian theology can make to our understanding of human rights in relation to HIV and AIDS. All three of them have made major personal contributions, over the years, to their churches' responses to AIDS. The Rev. Michael Schuenemeyer, executive director of the United Church of Christ AIDS programme in the USA, analyzes the undermining effects of a theological focus on sin upon a community's approach to human rights. The Rev. Ijeoma Ajibade, working with African communities in Britain, reflects on the relevance to her work of the idea of "imago Dei," the image of God. In South Africa, Dr Nontando Hadebe, teaching at a Catholic theological college in Johannesburg, turns to the theology of the Trinity for a rights-based model of community.

As we worked together on this book, we became aware that we were not able to include the full rich range of personal stories and insights that people brought to the table. To give some flavour of this richness we have included, at the beginning of each section, some of the thoughts and statements, many of them very personal, that people shared in the 2014 colloquium which gave a concrete shape to this publication. And because we hope that what we have done may be useable in parish or college settings, we have, at the end of each chapter, suggested a couple of questions with which readers might like to lead off their own discussions.

The final section has been coordinated by Lyn van Rooyen, director of CABSA (the Christian AIDS Bureau of Southern Africa). It opens with a special section devoted to essential reference material on the background to human rights, which would be invaluable for anyone wishing to make a serious study of the subject from an international perspective. We have, in addition, invited all the writers of this book to suggest accessible publications, links, and resources that offer valuable perspectives on HIV and human rights, in the hope that such a list may be of value to readers in their work.

Sin and fear

"You're going into the lions' den this time!" commented one colleague, when I said I had agreed to edit this book. "I hope you come out alive."

This is a difficult arena to enter, and she was only partly joking. The tendency to define HIV as a badge of immorality, not a communicable infection, has resulted in development of no-go areas in the discourse on HIV, and consequently increased the stigmatization and victimization of those affected. In these pages, especially in Part Two, there are many contextual examples. But as we write, the particularly sensitive no-go areas in the rights-versus-faith debate are those that relate to sexuality and sexual orientation. We should be deeply concerned that, in some parts of the world, men who have sex with men live in fear of being criminalized, hunted, beaten, or killed by people who believe the outlawing of gay men is necessary in order to protect marriage and the family and to defend the morals of the community. Just what are their persecutors afraid of?

Now fear is something that characterizes the early days of any epidemic, and AIDS was no exception. People fear what they do not know. Since then, over the years, public education has reduced (though not dispelled) the more irrational fears. But still, in terms of human rights, leaders are afraid that if they offer sanctuary to women and girls who are inappropriately pregnant, or if they accept the rights of gay men to live and love, then they are giving tacit approval to activities they believe to be immoral. So the theme of fear comes up again and again in these pages. And yet "Do not be afraid," or "Have no fear" are among the most frequently repeated instructions in our scriptures. We hear them from the angels who visit Zechariah, Mary and Joseph, from the shepherds in the fields on the night of Jesus' birth, and on numerous occasions in the course of his ministry. "Do not be afraid, little flock," he says, "for your Father has been pleased to give you the kingdom" (Luke 12:32).

So we do not need to be afraid. Honouring the rights of another does not mean I approve of what they do. It does not mean that I like them. Neither am I required to behave stupidly, and where there are rational grounds for taking suitable precautions, it is right to take them. What it does mean is that I recognize that we share a common humanity, and this means that whatever I think, or you think, we are, all of us, children of God, made in God's image, and as such we have, all of us, an inalienable right to be treated with dignity.

Questions for discussion

• Do you consider that human rights are an important issue in relation to HIV?

• Can you think of contexts in which it might be considered better to avoid talk of human rights?

Critical Issues

"Human beings have a God-given right to be."

"There is no point demanding your human rights if you are
alone on a desert island. Human rights only make sense as
a way of talking about what we owe to each other in our
common life together on this planet."
—Comments from participants in the 2014 colloquium

Part One of this volume consists of five chapters relating to issues that run
right through the response to HIV and AIDS: themes, indeed, that will appear
again and again in the pages that follow. Where do human rights come from,
and how do they interface with religion? When it comes to the response to HIV
and AIDS, what is it like to operate at the interface between human rights and
religion? Why is it so important that we understand and resist the destructive
power of stigma? Young women are exceptionally vulnerable to HIV: What
does it mean to claim that they have sexual and reproductive health rights, and
how can those rights be made a reality? And finally, since faith-related healthcare initiatives were often at the forefront of local and global responses to HIV,
we ask what are the particular challenges faced today by the many Christians
who are involved in the health sector.

Chapter 1

What's Wrong with Rights?

Julie Clague

You don't know what you are talking about!

What is a human right? We may think we know what we mean when we speak about human rights, but defining rights is tricky. Rights language is versatile, which means that rights can be invoked in a variety of ways to serve different purposes. The widespread use of rights language has made it a familiar, common currency in everyday life. However, generalized and unthinking appeals to rights have also led to a blurring of our concept of rights and a devaluing of its currency.

Human rights are essentially concerned with how people should be treated. They apply to all persons, wherever and whoever they are, solely by virtue of their being human. Yes, even the most "contemptible" and "worthless" individuals have human rights. In other words, despite all our differences (sex, religion, abilities, attributes, social roles, moral character, etc.), our common humanity puts us all on an equal footing in terms of our human rights. There is no point demanding your human rights if you are alone on a desert island. Human rights only make sense as a way of talking about what we owe to each other in our common life together on this planet. Human rights provide a way of speaking about the essential social conditions that are required for people to live a life that is dignified. Rights express the degree of protection that persons can expect from society, and the degree of freedom they can exercise. Their absence creates human misery, injustice, and social unrest. Rights are opposed to inhumane treatment and demeaning, undignified living conditions. When human rights are denied, justice demands that they be restored.

How many human rights are there?

Humankind's thinking about rights has evolved. The first generation of rights – articulated at the time of the English, American, and French Revolutions – comprised political and civil rights, such as the right to free speech and the right not to be tortured. They require the state not to interfere with their citizens. Since then, most nations have enacted laws to guarantee these political and civil rights. The second generation of rights was economic, social, and cultural in focus, including the right of all citizens to education, health care, and employment, reflecting the socialist insights of theorists such as Karl Marx. These second-generation rights require the state to engage actively in the delivery of essential services. The third generation of rights concerns the basic necessities of life, such as the right to food, water, and shelter. These third-generation rights can only be realized if there is a global effort to achieve an equitable distribution of resources. It is too big a challenge for any one nation.

Over time, the number and types of human rights have increased. Some are easily enshrined in law, others are not. Some are readily attainable; others remain aspirational. Would you like to see a definitive list of human rights? The key document is the 1948 Universal Declaration of Human Rights (UDHR). Since 1948, various other human rights instruments (e.g., covenants and conventions) have spelled out in more detail the nature of the rights contained in the Declaration. However, not all nations have signed up to all aspects of these various human rights documents. At the international level and at the grassroots level, people continue to debate and dispute the meaning and scope of certain rights. Article 3 of the Declaration states, "Everyone has the right to life." But how should this right be applied in practice? Should this include the unborn? Should this rule out the use of the death penalty by nation states? Article 16 includes the right to marry and to found a family. A small and growing number of nations regard this right as applying to same-sex couples. These examples show that while, in general terms, there is widespread international consensus about the importance of respecting the human rights listed in the Universal Declaration, there are also areas of continuing debate, disagreement, and evolution in humankind's thinking about human rights in practice.

Might is right

Human rights as we know them today came to prominence in the aftermath of the Second World War, as the world came to terms with the Nazi extermination programme that slaughtered Jewish citizens and other minority groups. Integral to the philosophy behind the foundation of the United Nations (UN) was the need to protect those who are treated with contempt, exploited or ignored by those in power. The UN Charter (1945) states: "The Purposes of the United Nations are: . . . promoting and encouraging respect for human rights and for fundamental freedoms for all without distinction as to race, sex, language, or religion." In the case of the Nazi holocaust, the atrocities committed were recognized by all to be utterly immoral crimes against humanity. This worldwide consensus allowed nations and peoples of widely differing, even opposed, world-views and philosophies to respond by signing up to a common code of practice – the above-mentioned UDHR – based upon universal standards of behaviour between states and their citizens, and between the citizens themselves. It states: "Recognition of the inherent dignity and of the equal and inalienable rights of all members of the human family is the foundation of freedom, justice and peace in the world."

God gave the Israelites rules for living in the form of the Ten Commandments. The UDHR summoned the nations of the world to agree upon a set of commitments to which others could hold them to account, and they created a supra-national mechanism of enforcement in an attempt to prevent further crimes against humanity. This does not mean human beings have changed: like Pharaoh of old, the powerful, wanting to preserve the status quo and retain power, continue to perpetrate or turn a blind eye to human rights abuses. Today, however, human rights do provide an international standard, independent of and superior to the laws of nations, by which wrongdoing, abuses of state power and unjust laws can be judged, and perpetrators held to account. The international community can appeal to international law based upon human rights norms and, through the UN, it can threaten sanctions to promote compliance by nation states.

Godless rights?

Most people on earth believe in God (or a god), but not everyone. Early drafts of the UDHR include explicit mention of God, as do the American Declaration of Independence (1776) and the French Declaration of the Rights of Man and of the Citizen (1789). In the final stages of drafting, however, references to God were removed from the text in the interests of garnering universal support and in order to avoid framing the UDHR in terms alien to non-believers. Clearly, the concept of human rights is a modern invention. You will not find human rights mentioned in the Bible.

But that doesn't invalidate them for believers. By the same token, you will not find mention of the Holy Trinity in the Bible. The Trinity is a concept that developed two centuries after the New Testament was written, in order to make sense of the biblical witness about the nature of the Godhead. The Trinity is a fundamental pillar of Christianity, even though the development of the theology of the Trinity occurred in the post-biblical era of the early church. Christians do not reject the theology of the Trinity on the grounds that it is non-biblical. Rather, Christians accept the theology of the Trinity because they regard it as being the fruit of the Bible. Nor should Christians dismiss human rights on the grounds that they are non-biblical. Indeed, many Christians see a strong correspondence between the rules for living found in the Bible and those proclaimed in the UDHR, with some arguing that the modern conception of human rights is a direct descendent of the biblical vision of how humans should treat one another. It is just, they say, that the language used is different. The Bible is in fact overflowing with concern for the needy, vulnerable, marginalized, and oppressed, and it contains a powerful critique of those who exploit others. It states that the community as a whole has a duty of care for those who have no one to look after them, such as widows and orphans. Neighbours – even enemies – should be treated as you yourself would wish to be treated. Most Christians have embraced human rights language as an alternative way of expressing the age-old wisdom and truth found in scripture. To the extent that human rights presuppose the inherent dignity, value, and worth of persons, expose unjust social arrangements, and provide a critique of human beings' inhumanity to other humans, they should be viewed as entirely compatible with Christianity.

Divine law and social order

The 19th-century hymn *All Things Bright and Beautiful*, by Mrs Cecil Alexander, contains the following verse, though it is often (not surprisingly) omitted from modern hymnbooks:

The rich man in his castle,
The poor man at his gate,
God made them high and lowly,
And ordered their estate.

This verse reveals a Christian attitude, widespread at the time, that assumes a God-given social order, hierarchical in character, in which each knows their place, performs certain social roles, enjoys certain role-differentiated privileges, and defers to authorities such as the church and the state. According to this view, the class-based social hierarchy was a given: an instance of God's ordering of the cosmos visible in nature's observable laws. Other supposedly natural and observable phenomena included the existence of a weaker sex and the division of humanity into advanced and primitive peoples. At one time, the church cited this divinely ordained natural order to condone the African slave trade and the subordination of wives to husbands.

Take slavery. Article four of the UDHR prohibits slavery. Today, the inhumanity of slavery is widely recognized. Yet, for most of human history, societies were built around slave ownership. There was a time, not so long ago, when Christians regarded slavery as morally permissible. Indeed, the Bible (including Jesus) takes slavery for granted. The first article of the UDHR proclaims, "All human beings are born free and equal in dignity and rights." Yet, in 1948, African Americans, descendants of victims of the slave trade, were treated as second-class citizens in the United States of America. While many American Christians were active in the civil rights movement of the 1950s and 1960s, campaigning to win equality for African Americans, others harboured white supremacist opinions antithetical to the gospel and the UDHR.

The world has also moved slowly in relation to the role of women. By the end of the Second World War many nations were extending suffrage to their women citizens and granting females employment rights and other privileges formerly granted only to males. Nonetheless, in 1948 when the UDHR was formally adopted, despite the reference in article 21 to "universal and equal suffrage" as the only acceptable basis for democratic elections, over one hundred nations had still not granted women the right to vote and stand in elections. We are heirs to an ambivalent human (and Christian) history. Gradually, however, humanity (including Christianity) has come to recognize that the differential treatment of certain groups on the grounds of their race, sex, or religion is unjust discrimination, opposed to human dignity. Nevertheless, to this day many Christians around the world invoke the Bible and God's law of nature to defend male superiority and the practice of wives submitting to their husbands. There is still a long way to go before Christians everywhere unanimously proclaim and promote the fundamental equality of humans.

Rights in conflict

It would be naïve, therefore, to imagine that human rights are non-controversial. In practice, there are deep ideological and moral disagreements about rights language. One of the difficulties involves the occasions when rights come into conflict. Human rights are frequently described as universal, indivisible, and inalienable. Yet, in a world of limited resources, not all rights can necessarily be satisfied. Education spending may give way to healthcare spending, or healthcare budgets may be squeezed by defense spending. The right to free speech may be curtailed when it is used to incite hate crimes that threaten the right to security of a minority. For authorities, the task – in the interests of the common good – is to make a judgment call between conflicting rights. But this is no easy task, especially where societies aim to maximize the degree of freedom of their citizens, and only limit some freedoms in order to better promote other fundamental freedoms. This is part of the give and take of social living. Citizens will willingly give up certain freedoms in the knowledge that they and others will gain in other respects.

However, it is more problematic when one group is expected to give so that another group can take, as can happen when the rights of a minority are curtailed in the interests of the majority. Between 1986 and 1989, when HIV and AIDS first became a public health threat in Cuba, the country operated a compulsory quarantine regime to separate and treat infected persons. This limitation on freedom of movement was widely criticized as an infringement of the rights of those infected with HIV. Other controversial instances of human rights being denied because of HIV include the compulsory testing of certain social groups, such as employers requiring personnel to undergo HIV tests, as happened when the Catholic Church tested would-be candidates for the priesthood in certain high prevalence countries.

Another criticism of rights language is that its use can prolong and exacerbate rather than resolve disagreements and conflicts. Opponents in moral debates often appeal to rights to support and defend their positions, and this gives rise to competing claims in which one right is pitted against an opposing right, with no obvious means of resolving the argument. In the case of abortion, the right to life of the unborn is pitted against the woman's right to choose. In our contentious moral climate, there are many pressure groups appealing to rights to make their case. This has given rise to a cacophony of "rightsism," in which angry protesters assert their rights in order to win over public opinion. It sometimes appears as if those who shout loudest stand the greatest chance of success. In such a confused and antagonistic climate, the resolution of complex moral issues becomes difficult. Consequently, some would prefer to avoid rights-talk entirely in these debates, since it often appears to function as an assertion of will rather than providing support for a moral position.

Are rights too Western?

The drafting committee that worked on the text of the UDHR was composed of representatives from East and West, North and South. There was a genuine attempt to create a text that reflected a broader intellectual and philosophical palette than Western ideas alone; one that could be owned by all people. Nevertheless, it is often remarked that because human rights are Western in their inspiration, they promote Western moral assumptions that do not translate well to non-Western contexts. In identifying the rights tradition as a Western invention, the universal applicability of the UDHR is called into question.

What, precisely, is meant by describing human rights as "Western"? This label usually denotes more than the provenance of the idea of rights. It signifies a package of features – regarded by some as undesirable – concerning the nature of the person and the nature of society. The Western concept of *the person* is, typically, the autonomous individual, whose self-interest leads to an assertion of rights claims over and against other members of society. The Western concept of *society* is frequently characterized as a consumer society comprising private individuals only loosely connected to one another. Accordingly, the Western concept of rights comes to be seen as individualistic and self-seeking. The growth of the consumer society has created a frenzy of rights claims by individuals interested in extracting from society what they are owed, without a corresponding sense of social responsibility and concern for the rights and freedoms of others.

It should be said that there is some truth to this characterization. However, it would be quite wrong to regard the whole of Western culture as individualistic, selfish, and lacking in social responsibility, just as it would be false to portray non-Western cultures as entirely composed of selfless communities united in observation of their social responsibilities. Nonetheless, the critique of rights as individualistic is a powerful one, first developed by Karl Marx in the 19th century. Marx recognized that there had been a shift away from an earlier conception of society where the focus was on not individual rights but social duty. Each person fulfilled the particular roles and duties of his or her station in life and, by so doing, the overall good of society was promoted. Disturbance of this social order, by a failure to perform one's proper role and responsibilities, leads to chaos. The give and take of social life is undermined when everyone takes and no one gives.

It was not only atheistic communists such as Marx who saw the negative consequences of unbridled individualism. Many churchgoers also regarded rights-based individualism as selfish and disruptive of the social order, and with the decline of Christianity in the West, it became possible to characterize Western individualism as a secular disease leading to moral decline. This, of course, was too reductive. Nevertheless, the idea of rights as a secular creed has gained support since the founding of the UN. In part this is because the UN must represent the interests of all peoples, whether religious or not, and the UDHR has taken on a quasi-religious significance as sacred text for this secular organization. It is also because, for non-believers and liberals, human rights can be utilized to critique the morally and socially conservative conception of society promoted by some strands of the church and other religious groups.

Rights-based thought proclaimed that all persons were equal. Yet, evidently, some were still more equal than others. In the supposedly "divinely ordained" social order, not everyone flourished. Society still tended to favour the rich and powerful. For others there were social costs, as the masses were put to work to benefit the few. During the 19th and 20th centuries, disadvantaged groups that had been denied their rights began to claim them. Workers campaigned for workers' rights. The women's movement campaigned for women's rights. The civil rights movement campaigned for African American rights. The gay liberation movement sought rights for homosexuals. Gradually, laws were changed to promote social inclusion and better reflect the diverse and multi-cultural nature of modern societies. At the international level, Asian and African colonies, which claimed the right to be free of their colonizers, sought and gained independence.

Not everyone has welcomed all these changes, however. For instance, Christianity remains divided about gay rights and, to a lesser degree, women's rights. In part, this is due to the biblical legacy. It is also because some Christians regard such rights as subversive of the social order and especially undermining of marriage and family life. In non-Western contexts, where family ties are the bedrock of a communitarian form of social life, and personal morality has not been privatized to the extent it has in the West, matters of gender and sexuality remain centrally important in the construction of social meaning and identity. In such contexts, the changing status of women and the freeing of conventions concerning sexuality can seem like a form of cultural imposition of Western immorality.

The UN – which has as its *raison d'être* the promotion of human rights – is often regarded as party to this "invasion" of Western values. The much-more-complex truth is that in tackling public health emergencies such as the HIV epidemic, where sexual transmission is a route of infection, the mixture of religion, rights, and morality creates a complicated and sometimes dangerous ideological cocktail that can increase stigma and discrimination as well as boost infection rates. One of the aims of this publication is to bring together the voices of individuals who are struggling to prevent that from happening, and to prove that human rights are indeed compatible with the Christian vision of the person and society.

Questions for discussion

- Have you encountered a situation in which rights seem to conflict with each other? Was this situation resolved, and if so, how satisfactory was the outcome?

- Which do you think are more important, individual rights or the rights of the wider community? Have you encountered examples of such a conflict?

Chapter 2

Part of the Solution *and* Part of the Problem?

Sally Smith

Reflections on standing in the gap

In 2004, I joined the staff of UNAIDS, and three years later – in 2007 – was appointed to the position of Community Mobilization Adviser for Partnership with Faith-based Organizations. Before this, through the 1980s and 1990s, I had worked as a nurse with a faith-based organization in Nepal, focusing on sexual and reproductive health and HIV.[1] So the whole of my professional experience has, broadly, involved standing in the gap between different worldviews, occupied with brokering dialogue and understanding between, on the one hand, the values of religious faith, and on the other, the values of human rights and principles of best medical practice in the field of sexual and reproductive health. The relationship is not an easy one; nevertheless, in this increasingly polarized field, I have learned some essential lessons in navigation, advocacy, translation, and negotiating. FBOs are definitely a part of the solution to ending the AIDS epidemic as a public health threat, but for many people living with HIV and key populations at greater risk of HIV, they are also part of the problem.

Inevitably, it has been a vital part of my own work to underline the importance of faith in the HIV response, and the common ground between human rights, evidence-informed medical practice, and the theological concepts of justice and dignity: a task in which I stand together, today, with a growing body of professional opinion. For example, the medical journal *The Lancet*, in the Executive Summary to its landmark series on faith-based health care,[2] reminds us that an estimated 84% of the world's population is religiously affiliated. "Faith," it says, "is a powerful force in the lives of individuals and communities worldwide. Citing geographical coverage, influence, and infrastructure, *The Lancet* series argues that building on the extensive experience, strengths, and capacities of faith-based organizations offers a unique opportunity to improve health outcomes.

Looking back in time to 1948, when the Universal Declaration of Human Rights (UDHR) was drafted, the UN engaged in discussion with religious communities and leaders from many faiths, who drew on important theological teaching and principles from within their own faith traditions. There is much common ground between human rights and the theological concepts of human dignity and justice.

In Geneva, in 2012, Archbishop Rowan Williams gave a public lecture on human rights and religious faith. Stressing the strong links that unite the two discourses, and the crucial importance to these links for the HIV response today, Williams called on the faith community to stay engaged in this debate. He said, "It is important for the language of rights not to lose its anchorage in a universal religious ethic – and just as important for religious believers not to back away from the territory and treat rights language as an essentially secular matter, potentially at odds with the morality and spirituality of believers."[3]

Why HIV exposes fault-lines in our societies

In 2015, I was co-author to an article in the *Lancet* series, mentioned earlier, entitled "Controversies in Faith and Health Care." This article provided the opportunity to look a bit more closely at some of these controversies in the light of the questions we are addressing in this book. HIV exposes human rights abuses in ways that no other condition does today. It makes us face up to contradictions (fault-lines) in our societies and faith communities. Because of HIV, families have rejected their loved ones, men have divorced their wives, and institutions have denied people health care, housing, and employment. Children have been excluded from school, people have been buried alive, or left unburied. Some churches, especially in the early days of this epidemic, prevented people living with HIV from getting married, being ordained, running the

Sunday school, or taking communion. Whilst there has been much progress, some of the attitudes behind these acts of discrimination still exist. Why is this?

The first reason is the enduring experience of stigma. In Chapter 3, Suzette Moses Burton of the Global Network of People Living with HIV or AIDS (GNP+) describes the development of the "People Living with HIV Stigma Index." An invaluable research tool, designed and led by people living with HIV, the Stigma Index records their experiences of abuse by measuring the stigma and discrimination they face in different parts of the world. The evidence from this research has proved to be a powerful tool in starting dialogue and in changing local and national policy and practices that negatively affect people living with HIV.

For example, on average one in eight people living with HIV report being denied health services and one in nine is denied employment; an average of 6 percent reported experiencing physical assault as a result of their HIV status. In response, initiatives such as the INERELA+ "SAVE" approach and the EAA Framework for Dialogue have made important strides in addressing stigma in faith communities. The Ecumenical HIV initiative in Africa has developed a range of theological materials to provide a solid foundation for non-discriminatory approaches to people living with HIV. UNAIDS has partnered with them to apply these approaches in a number of countries.

Secondly, the widespread influence of patriarchy in religious tradition is another, long-standing fault-line in many societies and religions: one that is exposed by lessons, coming from the HIV epidemic, about the negative impact of patriarchal attitudes and relationships on HIV-prevention programmes. Take, for example, the theological discourses that foster male dominance and pave the way for violence toward women and sexual minorities. Theologians from the African Circle of Concerned Women Theologians have done much important work on introducing an alternative discourse and unpacking some of the biblical narratives on rape and sexuality and the transformative approaches to masculinities.

Some groups interpret moral and religious teachings around sexual behaviour and marriage, along with some more exclusive concepts of church, in ways that are so idealized that they rarely exist in the real world, and meanwhile ignore the realities of many people's lives, both before marriage and after it. In some narratives the word "choice" becomes polarized to refer only to sexual orientation or abortion while ignoring the situation of the vast majority of young women, especially in the southern hemisphere, who have no choice as to who they marry, have sex with, or when they have children. When this happens, church teaching may become blind to the lived realities of their members, and the right to protect oneself from sexual infection becomes in itself a sin.

This critical fault line – namely the belief, in many parts of the world, that women, especially adolescent girls, do not have the right to a say in when, where, or with whom they have sexual relations or get married – does not just deny women the right to influence decisions about how to space or otherwise plan their families; it also removes their ability to protect themselves from HIV and other sexually transmitted infections. The particular challenges facing young women and girls, and the way they can be helped to understand and confront them, are discussed by World YWCA's Hendrica Okondo in Chapter 4.

What we do know, today, is that in Africa HIV infection rates are soaring among this group of young women and violence against women is routine in many parts of the world. Although women globally represent 50 percent of all adults living with HIV, in Sub-Saharan Africa (the most affected region) 59 percent of all those affected are women. AIDS is still the leading cause of death among women of reproductive age. In Southern and Eastern Africa, adolescent girls are infected five to seven years earlier than their male counterparts, and the prevalence of HIV infection among them is up to five times higher. Up to 45 percent of adolescent girls report that their first sexual experience was forced. Young women who experience intimate partner violence are 50 percent more likely to acquire HIV than women who have not.[4]

Adding insult to injury, some religious leaders will blame young women who report rape, berating them for wearing modern clothing and yet remaining silent on the sexual harassment and abuse they face from men in their community on a daily basis. These kinds of glaring inconsistencies continue to fuel heated debates on the use of condoms and on sexual education in schools. They have also led to controversy, contradiction, and polarization both within religious traditions and between faith-inspired groups and other actors in the response to HIV. The "We Will Speak Out" Coalition is one initiative that has made some important strides in countering some of these abuses, speaking out against sexual violence and creating safe spaces for survivors in faith communities.[5]

Thirdly, "raid and rescue" approaches to HIV arising from some interpretations of "salvation" can be problematic, for example: when they influence the program design of work with children or sex workers. Children have been some of those most left behind in the HIV response, whether they are affected by HIV themselves or orphaned in the sense that they have lost one or more parents to the epidemic.[6] In 2009, in *Home Truths: Facing the Facts on Children, AIDS, and Poverty*, the Joint Learning Initiative (JLICA) on Children and HIV report made strong policy recommendations on best practice for children affected by HIV. The JLICA report stressed the principle that the rights and interests of children are best served within communities, and within some kind of family structure. Three broad policies will make an immediate and long-lasting difference for children: first, supporting children through immediate or extended families and delivering integrated family-centred services; second, strengthening community action to support families; and third, addressing family poverty through national social protection.

In caring for the children of parents who have died of AIDS, many religious groups have made major contributions to the overall response to the epidemic. Faith-based organizations are doing excellent work placing children in need in extended families and communities and campaigning for affordable HIV medications suitable for children. On the other hand, the myth that most orphans and vulnerable children lack family and social networks has encouraged some authoritarian approaches to orphan-care, aimed at placing orphaned children in institutions, which are justified among some religious groups as exercises in "salvation." Sometimes referred to as "raid and rescue," the practice of "rescuing" children from familiar environments is, potentially, an abuse of rights. Children are best served by policies and programming that are responsive to the evidence, are AIDS-sensitive, and respect their rights.

Religiously justified "raid and rescue" attempts have also been aimed at sex workers, driven by the claim that these women or young men have been trafficked or otherwise forced into prostitution. It is important not to conflate trafficking and sexual exploitation with sex work. It is true that some women are victims of trafficking and have little or no ability to leave; some, however, enter sex work because of limited economic opportunities to earn a living wage.

Because sex work is posited as a valid occupation, activists reject both the ideology of "rescuing" women from prostitution and the human rights violations associated with coercive or moralistic programmes. They argue that money would be better spent on increasing sex workers access to justice, education, safe workplaces, finance, housing, health care and other building blocks of fulfilled lives.[7]

The issue of rights related to reproduction and sexual health is a complicated one, not least because it raises aspects of life and of relationships that are taboo in some cultures and, arguably, hard to discuss in all. Religious leaders themselves find this a difficult topic, particularly those who have grown up in patriarchal cultures and with patriarchal theological assumptions built into their understandings of institutional religion.

In recent years, some of the bitterest rights-related confrontations have been in the area of human sexuality and sexual orientation. Men who have sex with men and transgender people are at increased risk of HIV infection, and in countries where stigma towards LGBT people is high they find it difficult to access HIV prevention and treatment services. My work involves helping UNAIDS staff, faith-based health service providers, and men who have sex with men with advice and support in some of these highly charged and complex situations. For example, in 2013 a news item arrived on my desk from a UNAIDS country officer in Africa requesting help in responding to a situation involving the arrest of an AIDS activist, accused of being gay. Some religious leaders had recently encouraged the publication of an article in the national newspaper with the headline "Cage Filthy Homos," in which the author argued that homosexual people are "no better than dogs." This kind of language is completely unacceptable, highly stigmatizing, and damaging – such irresponsible media reporting can lead to violence toward people living with HIV and members of the lesbian, gay, bisexual, and transgender (LGBTI) community.

In Uganda, AIDS activist David Kato was killed following a similar exposé of gay AIDS activists by a national newspaper. When a retired Anglican Bishop reached out to provide spiritual support to LGBT people, he too became the target of hate attacks. In Nigeria, following the introduction of a bill criminalizing same sex activity in 2014, health workers providing HIV services to men who have sex with men were harassed and had to flee, leaving the clinic unattended. In both Uganda and Nigeria, however, faith-based healthcare providers have continued to strive, often in difficult circumstances, to provide confidential and non-judgmental HIV services to men who have sex with men.

In reviewing these human rights fault lines exposed by HIV, it seems to me that sensitivities around sexuality are among the most difficult issues we are facing in the health field today. Traditional interpretations of Christian, Islamic, and Jewish scriptures all claim that sexual activity should be limited to one man and one woman within the context of marriage, and that homosexual acts are not accepted. On the other hand, this contrasts with the lived experience of those many people who are lesbian, gay, bisexual, or transgendered, for whom this is not a lifestyle choice but an expression of their identity.

Importantly, many church leaders are prepared to speak out against violence, stigma, and discrimination toward LGBT persons. There are many religious leaders who are honestly grappling with these challenges and searching their own religious texts and teachings, reaching out to provide pastoral care and speaking out against sexual violence in all its forms. "If someone is gay and searches for the Lord and has good will," said Pope Francis in 2013, "then who am I to judge?"

UNAIDS offices have reached out to provide HIV services and support and refuge to men under attack, and have worked with supportive religious leaders to address the unacceptability of violence and with national authorities to repeal laws that are a hindrance to the HIV response. The following are some broad examples of UNAIDS partnerships with religious leaders and their initiatives on HIV.

The role of faith leaders in promoting human rights in the context of HIV

In recent years, despite the many controversies involved, faith leaders have played a crucial role in defending human rights, and UNAIDS has engaged in a range of activities to support this work. Examples include co-hosting a High-Level Religious Leaders Summit on HIV. As a result of this summit, more than 400 religious leaders have signed a commitment to action.[8] Follow up work has included a joint project between UNAIDS, the Ecumenical Advocacy Alliance, the Global Network of People Living with HIV and the International Network of Religious Leaders Living with and Personally Affected by HIV (EAA, GNP+ and INERELA+), to develop a Framework for Dialogue between religious leaders and networks of people living with HIV.

UNAIDS has engaged FBO health service providers in scaled-up treatment and prevention work. Current work includes efforts to document some of the good policy and practice in faith-based health care for HIV. From the earliest days of the epidemic, the church, and other faith-based organizations have been at the forefront of a caring response to people living with HIV. Today they remain one of the largest single providers of HIV-related care. Much of their work in this area is of high quality with impressive retention rates of people on antiretroviral medication, and there are strong examples of faith-based health service providers providing care without stigma and discrimination to everyone in need. This is hardly surprising: most religious traditions regard care for the sick, the most marginalized, and the vulnerable in society as being a virtue. The theological concepts of dignity, justice, solidarity, and subsidiarity underpin this approach, forming a strong basis for positive discussions with the human rights community.

UNAIDS has partnered with the We Will Speak Out Coalition and the UK government to address sexual and gender-based violence. This coalition has been working with religious leaders and communities to encourage them to speak out against sexual and gender-based violence and create safe spaces within faith communities for survivors.

Most recently UNAIDS has supported WHO and a range of FBO partners to build on the lessons learned from HIV in responding to the Ebola crisis. And – importantly – it has supported vital efforts to build a credible evidence base on religious and faith-based assets.

Ten years ago, there was deep skepticism within the UN system about the capacity of faith-based organizations to contribute positively to the response to HIV. Today, that is not the case. UN Secretary General Ban Ki Moon has established a United Nations Inter-Agency Task Force on Engaging Faith-based Organizations for the Millennium Development Goals, devoted to establishing synergies that will magnify this collaborative work. The Task Force is coordinated by UNFPA, who, in partnership with UNAIDS, has led some pioneering work to identify areas of synergy between faith communities and the challenges above around reproductive health.

UNAIDS Executive Director Michel Sidibé[9] and Deputy Executive Director Luiz Loures[10] have publicly recognized and supported this important work. UNAIDS has encouraged faith groups to develop theological reflection on HIV. This has included liturgies of lament, and also prayers and theologies of suffering that are designed to help those affected by HIV to face fear, sickness, and death and to accompany bereaved families through the loss of young people in the prime of their lives. We have seen faith leaders form partnerships across religious traditions to provide safe spaces for community dialogue on difficult and sensitive issues such as sexual transmission, death, gender inequality, human rights abuses, stigma, and discrimination. FBOs have cared for the sick, not just with practical care at home and in communities, but in terms of psychological and spiritual care that includes support through burial and bereavement. They have provided primary, secondary, and tertiary level professional health care through hospitals, clinics, and community health programmes. They have advocated powerfully for funding, for affordable pricing of medicines, for more attention to the needs of children living with HIV, and for policy and legal changes that will move the HIV response forward.

Bridging the gap: Joining with the voices of religious leaders in shaping policy

In September 2014, in parallel with the UN General Assembly in New York, UNFPA collaborated with UNAIDS to host a dialogue with religious leaders of all major faiths and from every continent. This resulted in a powerful call for world leaders to ensure stronger action on sexual health in the post-2015 development agenda and to challenge the use of religion as a reason to hold back progress on policy to address these critical issues. They struggled for two days with issues of content and wording. I will end with a quotation from the statement that emerged[11]:

> Not in our name should any mother die while giving birth. Not in our name should any girl, boy, woman or man be abused, violated, or killed. Not in our name should a girl child be deprived of her education, be married, be harmed or abused. Not in our name should anyone be denied access to basic health care, nor should a child or an adolescent be denied knowledge of and care for her/his body. Not in our name should any person be denied their human rights.
>
> We affirm that sexual and reproductive health are part of human rights, and as such, must be guaranteed by governments. We note in particular the importance of preventing gender-based discrimination, violence and harmful practices; upholding gender justice; ensuring that every pregnancy is wanted and that every birth is safe; providing age-appropriate sexuality education; promoting the health, education and participation of youth and adolescents; preventing, treating and caring for people with HIV/AIDS; supporting family planning; and respecting the human body.

Resources

Ecumenical Advocacy Alliance. http://www.oikoumene.org/en/what-we-do/eaa.

Ecumenical Advocacy Alliance. "Religious Leadership in Response to HIV." http://www.e-alliance.ch/en/s/hivaids/summit-of-high-level-religious/index.html.

Ecumenical HIV and AIDS Initiatives and Advocacy (EHAIA). https://www.oikoumene.org/en/what-we-do/ehaia.

"Faith Based Health Care." *The Lancet*, 7 July 2015. http://www.thelancet.com/series/faith-based-health-care.

Framework for Dialogue between Religious Leaders and People Living with HIV. http://www.frameworkfordialogue.net/.

JLIC. *Home Truths: Facing the Facts on Children, AIDS, and Poverty: Final Report of the Joint Learning Initiative on Children and HIV/AIDS* (2009). http://www.unicef.org/malaysia/JLICA_-_2009_-_Home_Truths_Children_AIDS_poverty.pdf.

INERELA+ SAVE toolkit. http://inerela.org/resources/save-toolkit/.

People Living with HIV Stigma Index. http://www.stigmaindex.org/.

Marshall, Katherine, and Sally Smith. "Religion and Ebola: Learning from Experience." *The Lancet*, 6 July 2015. http://www.thelancet.com/journals/lancet/article/PIIS0140-6736(15)61082-0/abstract.

UNAIDS. *A Call to Action Faith for Sexual and Reproductive Health and Reproductive Rights Post 2015 Development Agenda*, 19 September 2014. http://www.unfpa.org/sites/default/files/resource-pdf/Faith%20leaders%27%20call% 20to%20action.pdf.

UNAIDS. *Gap Report* (2014). http://www.unaids.org/en/resources/campaigns/2014gapreport.

UNAIDS. *Guidance Note on Sex Work* (2013). http://www.unaids.org/sites/default/files/sub_landing/files/JC2306_UNAIDS-guidance-note-HIV-sex-work_en.pdf.

UNAIDS and Stop AIDS Alliance. *Communities Deliver* (2015). http://www.unaids.org/sites/default/files/media_asset/UNAIDS_JC2725_CommunitiesDeliver_en.pdf.

Question for discussion

- In your experience, what are the cross-cutting human rights issues that recur again and again as Christians and Christian organizations respond to HIV and AIDS?

Chapter 3

Why Stigma Matters

Suzette Moses-Burton

My faith is inextricably linked to who I am as a human being. It is the reason that I was able to defy the 'death sentence' of an HIV diagnosis in the early 90s. Without it, I would have no hope, no strength and no determination to live. Yet, as a Christian living with HIV, in a world filled with the insidiousness of HIV-related stigma, how do I reconcile my own view of my soul as black instead of the purity of white, when who I so often see in the mirror, is society's reflection of who I am as a person living with HIV, the sinner, and never the saint?

These are my own words: words I heard myself saying, one day, in one of the meetings that led to the creation of this book. Stigma is deeply personal. It does matter.

Here's why.

More than a third of Zambians living with HIV have experienced physical assault as a result of stigma surrounding the virus, and two out of five have lost their jobs. One in five Ukrainians and one in three Columbians living with HIV have been denied health care. One out of three Colombians and more than a quarter of Zambians have been excluded from family activities. One out of five Colombians and one out of seven Nepalese living with HIV have experienced suicidal feelings.

These are snapshots of the real and devastating impact that HIV-related stigma has on communities of people living with HIV around the world. They emerge from the Zambian, Ukrainian, Colombian, and Nepalese People Living with HIV Stigma Index.

Stigma may at first appear to be an abstract concept: but every statistic points to such disturbing individual stories of personal frustration and despair, of people ostracized by friends, family, schools, workplaces – and sadly, also the church and its congregations – just at a time when they most need support. Stigma hurts people. It affects quality of care, access to services, and support networks such as family, friends, and church. It impacts people's ability and willingness to start treatment, continue taking their treatment, and stay connected with clinics and other service providers.

Without action on stigma and the underlying factors that cause it, increased access to treatment alone will not be effective in bringing about the end to AIDS. Over the past 15 years, we have seen a significant increase in access to HIV treatment despite the challenges of limited access in many countries. So why is it that globally, in rich countries and poor, we still see people dying of AIDS? The answer, in many cases, is stigma – that little word that has such a major influence on how, why, where, and when people living with HIV access life-saving treatment, and also on their physical and emotional health and well-being. It is horrifying and unacceptable that in 2015 a virus that in clinical terms has progressed from being a death sentence to a chronic manageable disease remains so stigmatized in so many parts of the world.

Stigma – and its close cousin, discrimination – are widely recognized as barriers to prevention, treatment, care, and support; yet the global health system has focused very little attention on decreasing their impact, favouring instead other, more technical, solutions. The challenge seems to lie in the fact that global policy makers don't consider stigma to be sufficiently measurable, nor do they believe it can be changed through programmatic approaches. This is not only incorrect, but a dangerous and damaging assumption.

Stigma exists in many forms and has the effect of devaluing, demeaning, or discrediting individuals in the eyes of others. Stigma can be the *external stigma* that people living with HIV experience from other people, including insults, rejection, avoidance, intolerance, stereotyping, discrimination, or – even more odious – physical violence. Equally damaging, though less often heard or talked about, is *internalized stigma*: the negative thoughts and feelings about themselves that people living with HIV often experience, profoundly affecting how they live their lives or value themselves as human beings, and leading many to choose instead to live in isolation or fear, deliberately avoiding meaningful relationships with others. Thirdly, there also exists the *anticipation of stigma*, which may be closely related to internalized stigma. Fourthly, there are those who experience *stigma by association* because of their friendship, relationship, or other links with a stigmatized individual or group.

In considering all these factors we need, also, to view them in the context of problems that pervade countries where the epidemic is at its most concentrated: poverty, social inequality, gender-based violence, and cultural norms. Further, let us not forget that many people living with HIV may suffer multiple forms of intersecting stigma, and that these can compound feelings of isolation and marginalization. These include communities such as sex workers, people who use drugs, transgender persons, and men who have sex with men: groups that often have been forced to the edges of society, existing stigmatization being reinforced by discriminatory and punitive laws and policies. The church has too often played its role in contributing to the epidemic of HIV-related stigma, forgetting Christ's message of love, which lies at the heart of the bible and its teachings.

This is where the People Living with HIV Stigma Index comes in.[1] This is a research tool to measure stigma and discrimination as experienced by people living with HIV and to map where it occurs and how it is manifested, and so to contribute to the growing evidence base confirming fears about the extent of the problem. To date, more than 50 countries have implemented the People Living with HIV Stigma Index, over 1,300 people living with HIV have been trained as interviewers, and a further 45,000 people living with HIV have been interviewed. The Index tool contains a questionnaire and a user guide (translated into 54 languages), which supports networks of people living with HIV in conducting the research. It can easily be adapted by different groups of people living with HIV seeking to understand their experiences of stigma and discrimination in their local context.

The core value of the tool is that it is a participatory and interactive learning-by-doing model, upholding the GIPA principle (Greater Involvement of People Living with HIV and AIDS). Research is carried out *by* people living with HIV, *for* people living with HIV. The results are owned by the community that collected the data, empowering them and creating direct change within that community. The process of undertaking the research is, in many ways, just as important as the final results. The researchers build their capacity and research skills, and through the process, build their confidence to become advocates for the rights of people living with HIV. As members of the community of people living with HIV, they are in the best position to understand the daily challenges of living with HIV and how stigma affects them. In reaching out to and interviewing individuals, they play a role in connecting those people to a sense that they are part of a journey that is being walked by many individuals – not alone, but together – building a sense of solidarity and community.

What this research achieves is to put evidence in the hands of networks of people living with HIV that enables them to advocate with their national governments. The impact of having such information available in a measurable form to present to policy makers is enormous, increasing understanding at all levels about how stigma and discrimination works and how it is experienced by people living with HIV, highlighting neglected areas requiring action, and shaping future programmatic interventions and policy changes. These might include improved workplace policies, more informed debates about the criminalization of HIV transmission, and promotion of human rights.

There is much evidence that this works. In Kenya, Ethiopia, and South Africa, the Stigma Index now forms part of their respective National HIV Strategic Plans and is being supported by their respective National AIDS Consortia. In South Africa, NAPWA (the national PLHIV network) partnered with Ekurhuleni Pride Organizing Committee (EPOC) to conduct advocacy using the evidence they gathered, leading to a stakeholders' meeting with Gauteng Provincial Government departments, human rights organizations, women's organizations, LGBTI organizations, PLHIV networks, traditional leaders, UN agencies, and representatives of government departments. This advocacy successfully enabled the LGBTI community representatives to have a position on the provincial AIDS council.

The evidence of the Stigma Index is also used as the basis for dialogues between religious leaders and networks of people living with HIV using the Framework for Dialogue methodology.[2] In Malawi, Ethiopia, Kenya, Uganda and other countries, these dialogues have led to collaborative efforts, such as workplace policies, sermon guides, training, to help reduce stigma and inspire joint advocacy between religious leaders and people living with HIV.

Moreover, the results have been used in many cases to highlight the needs and experiences of marginalized groups, such as men who have sex with men (MSM), who are often hidden and difficult to reach. Having evidence can help to create a space for dialogue that didn't previously exist. In Malawi, members of the national network of people living with HIV used evidence from the Stigma Index to engage with parliamentarians on MSM issues. These parliamentarians are now becoming increasingly open to dialogue and have spoken of the need to ensure that treatment is accessible for all who need it. In Tanzania, for the first time, the evidence of the Index led to the National Strategic Plan containing specific reference to the needs of key populations. In Senegal, it led to the first-ever public rally in support of the rights of people living with HIV, including MSM. In 2008, Senegalese MSM were not welcome as members of the national people living with HIV network, but now there are MSM members on the board and in the network. These examples are just some of the many that show how crucial it is to develop tools that enable people living with HIV to advocate for real change in their countries, and what a profound effect it can have in changing national debate and dialogue around the issue.

Significantly, we need to understand that action on stigma is often most effective when people living with HIV lead it. That is why funding for civil society, and particularly for networks of people living with HIV at national and regional levels, needs to be a core component of the HIV response, particularly as we enter into the post-2015 era of the Sustainable Development Goals. Policy-makers need to recognize that far from being a "fuzzy" solution to ending AIDS, direct funding to communities of people living with HIV has a proven and measurable impact on the course of the epidemic. We have never been the problem, but an integral part of the solution. There should be nothing for us, without us.

The brutal murder of HIV activist Gugu Dlamini in KwaMashu in South Africa, who spoke out and publicly disclosed her HIV status in 1998, is the most heinous form of HIV-related stigma. But let's not also forget those quieter and less-publicized deaths – people who commit suicide rather than suffer the shame they feel around their diagnosis; people who suspect they know their status, but choose instead to live in denial until they are so ill that they cannot be saved; people who sit quietly and largely unnoticed in congregation pews, desperately seeking salvation and acceptance as bible-thumping pastors rain hell fire and brimstone down on them instead; people, who because of the shame of their families or the discrimination of healthcare workers, don't access the life-saving treatment or care that they need; marginalized people who are also criminalized. These are also the people who are killed by stigma, and they are dying in the thousands.

For them, we need to take action on stigma NOW!

Resources

Gideon Byamugisha's publications for Strategies for Hope. These include *Open Secret: People Facing up to HIV and AIDS in Uganda* (2000); *Journeys of Faith: Church-based Responses to HIV and AIDS in Three Southern African Countries* (2002), and *Positive Voices: Religious Leaders Living with or Personally Affected by HIV and AIDS* (2005).

Paterson, Gillian. *Aids Related Stigma: Thinking Outside the Box – The Theological Challenge*. Geneva: EAA, 2005. http://www.e-alliance.ch/en/s/hivaids/stigma/aids-related-stigma-resource/index.html.

Paterson, Gillian. "HIV, AIDS and Stigma: Discerning the Silences." In B. Haddad, *Religion, HIV and AIDS: Charting the Terrain*. University of Kwa-Zulu Natal Press, 2011.

People Living with HIV Stigma Index. http://www.stigmaindex.org/.

Questions for discussion

- Have you ever been at the receiving end of stigma? How did it feel? Were you discriminated against in concrete ways? Return now to Suzette's words in the opening paragraph of this chapter, and comment on how they make you feel.

- Have you yourself ever refused to be with someone, denied help, talked disparagingly about someone whether they were present or not – because there was something that made them different or made you uncomfortable? At the time, how did you justify this to yourself? Would you act any differently now?

Chapter 4

Sexual and Reproductive Health Rights for Young Women

Hendrica Okondo

What has been agreed internationally

In 1979, the United Nations' (UN) General Assembly adopted the Convention on the Elimination of All Forms of Discrimination against Women (CEDAW), which recognized the sexual and reproductive health rights of girls and women. The convention's various articles are designed to protect girls' and women's right to equal access to reproductive health services and offer protection from all forms of abuse, including physical, mental, and sexual abuse. CEDAW also promotes girls' and women's right to seek and receive accurate information on their sexual and reproductive health.

In 1994, at the International Conference on Population and Development in Cairo (ICPD), UN member states took this further, agreeing to put human rights at the heart of all development interventions. This, it was believed, would improve the quality of life for all individuals, securing their potential by eliminating all institutional barriers that promote discrimination, particularly in relation to women and girls.

In 2012, in Bali, Indonesia, the UN mobilized young people to review the earlier ICPD Programme of Action. Resolutions from the Bali meeting recommended interventions that would protect the rights of adolescents and youth to exercise control over their bodies, and to decide freely and responsibly on matters relating to their sexuality, regardless of age and marital status. This would include sexual and reproductive health.

In 2014, UN agencies launched a global review of the Beijing Platform for Action on women's rights, and of the ICPD Programme of Action. The outcome was a paper urging governments and agencies to promote equality by tackling the structural inequalities in societies that place limitations on the ability of their citizens to exercise their sexual and reproductive rights. One of these rights was universal access to available, accessible, acceptable, high quality, comprehensive, and integrated sexual and reproductive health information and services for all their people. In resonance with CEDAW, the Beijing +20 review outcome has particularly underscored the need to pay attention "to the health education of adolescents, including information and counseling on all methods of family planning." It further specified that health education for adolescents should address "gender equality, violence, prevention of sexually transmitted diseases and reproductive sexual health rights."

The way it really is

Reading through these global protocols, one might come away with the impression that the struggle for young women's health rights is won. However the reality is, all too often, that adolescent girls and young woman are prevented from exercising rights by the prevalence of unequal power structures and harmful traditional practices. Globally, since the year 2000, over 67 million girls and young women have been forced into marriage, mostly before age of 15 years. These girls are denied the basic right to education, the right to choose their partner, and the right to health care. In many regions they are subjected to harmful traditional practices, such as female genital mutilation, traditional sexual initiation, coercion, and sexual abuse. Yet they face legal, cultural, and religious barriers preventing them from accessing the sexual and reproductive health information and services which (according to the above conventions, and often agreed to by their own governments) are their legal right.

In Africa, the World YWCA runs "safe space" programmes in its 28 member associations. Africa has the worst indicators, with 16 million girls married annually before the age of 18. Of the 20 countries with the highest prevalence of child, early, and forced marriages, 15 are in Africa. In order to secure marriages for these young women, many communities will condone harmful practices such as breast massaging, abduction, rape, and widow cleansing. Three million girls in sub-Saharan Africa undergo FGM/C (female genital mutilation or cutting): a blatant a violation of their rights, yet considered a key practice in ensuring sexual purity before marriage.

Girls who marry early are at high risk of HIV infection, many of them having no knowledge of how HIV is transmitted, no capacity to negotiate for protection with partners who are older, and limited agency to make sexual and reproductive health decisions. It is important to understand the link between denial of the sexual and reproductive health rights of these girls and young women and the high level of HIV infection rates among them. Sexually transmitted diseases increase the risk of acquiring and transmitting HIV, especially where young women are forcibly married or forced by poverty into transactional sexual activities with older men. Hence AIDS-related illnesses are a leading cause of maternal death in young women, accounting for 13 percent of the deaths of pregnant girls in Africa.

Sadly, knowledge about HIV among women below the age of 25 years and adolescent girls has increased painfully slowly, standing now at 34 percent, well behind the UNGASS 2015 target of 95 percent. It is therefore not surprising that the estimated number of HIV-positive adolescent girls and young women is rising. In Tanzania, Kenya, and Zambia, prevalence rates among young women are 4.1 percent, 3.9 percent, and 8.9 percent respectively: that is, approximately eight times higher than that of their male peers.

Faith communities are involved

Despite this overwhelming evidence, many faith leaders continue to support parents and guardians who are intent on forcing adolescent girls and young women into early marriage. Many faith communities are modeled on hierarchy and patriarchy, where the father or male guardian has the last word. The subordination of girls and women is often justified by religious texts such as, for example, "I want you to understand that the head of all humanity is Christ and the head of the wife is her husband" (1 Cor. 11:3a NIV). In many faith communities in Africa, this is translated to mean that every girl and women has, over her, a male authority figure, and all male authority is guided and authorized by Christ. This means that men's decisions are from God: a belief that is often exaggerated if the authority in question is a religious leader. Abuse by families may be legitimized when girls and women have to obey the instructions of this male leader: obedience that often is equated to the obedience to God.

Yet we also know faith can be a liberating force for girls and women. Working with female theologians, the World YWCA has begun to move beyond cultural constraints in interrogating these Bible texts. We have noted that there are life-giving texts that affirm that all human beings are created in the image of God. Faith communities can be hope-sharing and care-giving spaces, giving us models of Christian community which support the belief that girls and young women can live fulfilled lives where they can access their right to education and health and achieve their full potential.

Sophia Chirongoma is a feminist theologian who works with the World Council of Churches' EHAIA initiative. Participating in a regional training programme for World YWCA members in Arusha, Tanzania, Sophie argued that young women and men of faith are called to disrupt these negative practices and promote a biblical image of equality and justice. Justice, she stressed, means opportunities for all, pointing to a need for constant dialogue and advocacy in order to create a platform for engaging religious leaders and sharing insights with them. For the truth is that some of them do not have the necessary tools and skills to address this major crisis of child marriage, early marriage, and forced marriage, and find themselves conflicted by the theological struggles on such sensitive subjects. For example, they do not know how to challenge parents who believe that when they force a girl to marry her rapist, they are protecting their child from shame; or they believe that when they send away pregnant girls, they are saving them from social stigma.

What we can do to help

The World YWCA has addressed these challenges by developing "Safe Spaces for Women and Girls: A Global Model for Change." Here the girls are made aware of their rights with the help of a network of peer educators who have experienced the abuse. It is their job to mobilize groups of young women, who become safe-space leaders for collective action when one of them is married off. Meanwhile, leading advocacy campaigns at national, regional, and global levels ensure girls in marriage, or at risk of marriage, have access to legal support, education, and health opportunities that will ensure an economic livelihood.

Training of trainers has been organized in Africa in collaboration with EHAIA. These initiatives have provided space for dialogue and learning between religious leaders and young women, enabling them to interrogate traditions that continue to keep women and girls in situations that deny them access to sexual and reproductive health and rights: situations that compromise their decision-making processes and eventually expose them to the risk of HIV infection. Today, these dialogues have begun to address the silence surrounding issues to do with the sexuality of women and girls.

In our work in Africa we have encountered many young women who have suffered from abuse. One example is "Mary," a young woman who became a safe-space leader at one of our YWCA safe spaces in Zambia. Mary was frequently sexually harassed by a married man who was her teacher at school. When she described the harassment to her parents, they decided it was time for her to undergo a traditional initiation ceremony, which included being forced to have sex with an older man. Her mother had no say in the process: her father, a pastor, made all the arrangements. Within months she was pregnant, tested HIV positive, and was obliged to drop out of school. She was then forced to marry the teacher who had harassed her and who, by paying a fine, managed to avoid being reported to the authorities.

Mary had a second child with him before he was transferred to another district, leaving her with two children she could not care for. One died, leaving her with a daughter who was also HIV positive. Her participation in the YWCA safe space enabled Mary to go back to school, start on HIV treatment, and ensure that her daughter was treated. Her parents were reluctant to seek legal advice, so Mary never got justice for her case. Nevertheless, she became an active safe space leader and, in a district where young women have an HIV prevalence rate of 18.9 percent, she rescued many other girls who faced similar experiences.

Today, Mary works with traditional and religious leaders, using a human rights approach to reach out to communities. She is accompanied by a police officer from the Gender Support Unit and a religious leader who has been trained through the EHAIA programme. The team trains mothers, fathers, and other guardians in the family on the rights of young women and the importance of supporting them to stay in school or, if they become pregnant, to return to school. The team also ensures that perpetrators are punished when young girls become pregnant.

Mukatimui Sitali Indopu is the project director of this YWCA branch. In a recent presentation about this NORAD-funded project, he spoke about the human rights-based approach the programme uses in counteracting stigma and discrimination. This involves peer to peer counseling, home-based care and visits, appointment accompaniment for testing and care, and the training of teachers, traditional and faith leaders, and service providers. Due to demand, the programme has expanded to a peer education network of 67 female and 11 male workers, reaching out to 4000 women, young women, and girls, over 100 male leaders, and 500 young men. Mukatimui also described the follow-up support that the YWCA in Zambia promotes, stating, "Once these young women have recovered from their illness and self-stigmatization, they are encouraged to join a safe-spaces club where they can disclose their status without facing judgment, and get information on living positively and referrals to trained health workers." Today, this support has been expanded to involve economic empowerment, with young women being trained in business management. Some women in this programme started a poultry farm and were able to begin farming tomatoes and rice, supporting their nutritional needs as well as providing economic independence. In these ways, the targeting of young women's rights has become a key element in the struggle against HIV, not just for women and girls but for whole communities.

Resources

CEDAW. *The Convention on the Elimination of All Forms of Discrimination against Women.* http://www.un.org/womenwatch/daw/cedaw/.

World YWCA. *Safe Spaces for Women and Girls: A Global Model for Change.* http://www.worldywca.org/Resources/YWCA-Publications/YWCA-Safe-Spaces-for-Women-and-Girls-A-Global-Model-for-Change.

UN Women. *Step It up for Gender Equality: The Beijing Platform for Action Turns 20.* http://beijing20.unwomen.org/en/step-it-up.

Questions for discussion

- What explanation would you offer for the fact that young women are so vulnerable to HIV and AIDS?
- Are there parallels between your own context and the one Hendrica Okondo is describing?
- Does this qualify as a human rights issue, and if so, why?

Chapter 5

Health Care, HIV, and Human Rights: An Approach That Works

Callie Long

Why is there a problem?

In the late 1980s and 1990s, HIV cast a long shadow over the lives of millions of people. A common thread ran through the many responses to this new and frightening disease: the fact that in many parts of the world, it was the local faith-based communities who provided care and compassion to those who needed it the most.

This should not come as a surprise. Faith-based communities, organizations, and institutions have long been involved with health care through local outreach programs and interpersonal support at community level, as well as at mission hospitals and clinics. It was likely, therefore, that many would respond when HIV first began to take its toll. Faith-based groups with their roots in communities were trusted. They brought to the task their existing networks, communities of motivated people, and often some resources. Many tried hard to address the myths and misinformation that were so common in the early days of the epidemic, despite the fact that in doing so they often found themselves facing the fear, denial, stigma, and discrimination that HIV itself attracted.

In a perfect world, this would be the full faith-related story: a story of empathy, kindness, love, and resolve; of mobilizing scarce resources to engage with human tragedy. Sadly, though, the history of the epidemic also shows that religious convictions have been the grounds for condemnation, judgment, stigma, and rejection directed at people living with or affected by HIV. So responses were mixed; opportunities were missed. Taken together, these two narratives – the positive and the negative - have set the stage for deep ambivalence toward the faith-based communities' responses to HIV.

In my long-standing involvement with the global AIDS advocacy movement, I have found faith-based communities to be among the cornerstones of any commitment to prevention, care, and treatment. Although my own work is entirely secular, I have seen just how powerful a force faith can be and how deeply it can influence both health and behaviour.

I am also aware that faith-inspired activity is not always taken into account in public health discourses. Sally Smith, earlier in this book, referred to *The Lancet*'s Faith and Health Series (July 2015),[1] which set out some of the unique characteristics of faith-based health care. These, it is suggested, include "access to hard-to-reach populations, priority for poor and marginalized people, mobilization and support of volunteers, and innovative fee structures and governance approaches." The authors also list some of the disadvantages that occur, such as "inadequate or unpredictable financings, variable governance, or priorities and strategies that differ from national health systems." They refer to the ongoing debates between the many health professionals who have blamed religions for moralistic attitudes that undermine prevention efforts by encouraging stigma and denial: to which religiously motivated people may respond by blaming increases in new cases of HIV upon organizations that promote "liberal" approaches to sexuality, believing that these have led to a decline in morality and therefore an increase in HIV.

Human rights are not abstract

Human rights approaches to HIV are not abstract. Rather they are real, proven, practical, and cost-effective ways to address and respond to HIV. The joint statement *Human Rights: Now More Than Ever* was drafted initially for the 2006 International AIDS Conference and subsequently endorsed by hundreds of AIDS advocates. It demonstrates the determination of AIDS activists to place human rights at the centre of the global response. The protection of a full range of human rights, it says, is the key to protecting public health.

The Global Fund to Fight AIDS, Tuberculosis and Malaria deems certain groups of people as "key populations" if they meet all three of the criteria below:

Epidemiologically, the group faces increased risk, vulnerability and/or burden with respect to at least one of the three diseases – due to a combination of biological, socioeconomic and structural factors;

Access to relevant services is significantly lower for the group than for the rest of the population – meaning that efforts and strategic investments are required to expand coverage, equity and accessibility for such a group; and

The group faces frequent human rights violations, systematic disenfranchisement, social and economic marginalization and/or criminalization – which increases vulnerability and risk and reduces access to essential services.

—Key Populations Action Plan (2014-2017), www.theglobalfund. org/.../Publication_KeyPopulations_ActionPlan_en/

Human rights activists have achieved great gains in the response to HIV: the right to non-discrimination on the basis of HIV status; the right to treatment as part of essential health care; and the right of people living with HIV and AIDS to participate in the development of AIDS policies and programs.[2]

Countless examples bear witness to how these advocates – many from within the faith community – were among the first to highlight the importance of "increasing access to HIV testing as part of the right to the highest attainable standard of health."[3] In this task, they have been hindered by the fact that religiously motivated interventions have too often classified HIV as a moral condition instead of a medical one: a view that has had fatal consequences in contexts where seeking help is in itself an admission of "sin." To equate HIV and AIDS with sin and to judge or reject people on those grounds will only discourage them from accessing critical services. Worse, fear of condemnation may drive them underground, so that they will not go for testing, not seek treatment, and not take crucial steps to avoid transmission of the virus. Thus

"Rights-based" responses to HIV are practical, and they work. (From the Now More than Ever Campaign)

Human rights approaches to HIV are not abstract, but real, practical, and cost-effective. Countries that have placed human rights at the center of their AIDS responses have seen epidemics averted or slowed. Examples of human rights responses to HIV include the following:

1. Ensuring that national HIV programs include measures to combat discrimination and violence against people living with HIV or AIDS and those at risk of infection.
2. Ensuring that young people have full access to HIV information, sexual and life skills education, as well as to condoms and services for sexually transmitted infections and family planning.
3. Investing in legal empowerment of people living with HIV and AIDS so that they know their rights and can mobilize around them.
4. Making policy changes to reduce prison overcrowding so that people are not incarcerated illegally, and consequently less vulnerable to HIV from sexual violence and needle-sharing while incarcerated.
5. Removing legal and other barriers to evidence-based HIV prevention and treatment for people who use illegal drugs.
6. Establishing clear legal remedies for violence and discrimination against sex workers, men who have sex with men, transgender people, and other marginalized groups.
7. Providing women and girls with effective remedies against all forms of gender-based violence, inside and outside marriage, as well as redress against legally sanctioned discrimination in access to economic opportunities, property, and inheritance.

http://www.hivhumanrightsnow.org/10-reasons/
rights-based-responses/

much of the good work done by faith-based institutions over the decades is undone.

Who, then, are these people who are judged to be so unworthy of society's respect?

They are often people already sidelined and pushed to the edges. They are often sex workers, people who use drugs, gay men, and other men who have sex with men. A recent policy brief, *Transgender People and HIV*[4] (World Health Organization, July 2015), suggests that transgender women are disproportionately affected. All of them are people who are particularly vulnerable to HIV, and then face social marginalization, criminalization, and a range of other human rights abuses that increase their existing vulnerability to HIV.

Criminalization related to HIV status is becoming an increasingly serious threat to public health. According to the Global Fund to Fight AIDS, Tuberculosis and Malaria, at least 63 countries have jurisdictions with HIV-specific criminal statutes, 17 of which have prosecuted individuals under these laws. In 2000, no African country had an HIV-specific criminal statute. Today, says the Global Fund's Key Populations Action Plan (2014-2017), Africa has 27 countries with HIV-specific criminal statutes, followed by Asia (13), Latin America (11), and Europe (9).[5] Three examples from the report/plan starkly illustrate just how massive a barrier criminalization is to accessing healthcare provisions:

- In most of Eastern Europe and Asia, people who inject drugs face denial of health services, potential arrest, and harassment by police. Proven means of HIV prevention such as substitution therapy are illegal in many countries.

- In Russia, fewer than one in one hundred people living with HIV who inject drugs are receiving HIV treatment.

- In several countries of Southern Africa where homosexuality is criminalized, one in five men who have sex with men have reported being blackmailed because of their sexuality, and those experiencing blackmail have been less likely to seek health services.

Being a woman

Women are disproportionately affected by the epidemic. Just *being* a woman can increase one's vulnerability to HIV. The late Robert Carr was a long-time HIV advocate who dedicated his life to bringing attention to issues of

HIV-related stigma and discrimination. Here Carr summed up the discrimination women suffer simply by virtue of their gender:

> Whether as wives or mothers, as women who use drugs or as women who sell sex . . . women and girls, because of gender inequality and stereotypes, experience profound stigma. For example, women experience greater stigma for selling sex than men do for buying it – as it goes against ideas of women upholding societal virtues and needing to belong to one man. As a result, female sex workers are more likely to experience housing discrimination, violence, discrimination against their children and other forms of stigma. Across the board, we see stigma made worse by gender prejudices and the idea that a woman's biology sets her destiny. We will never make progress in the response to HIV – prevention, treatment, care, or support – unless we deal with the gender dimensions of HIV-related fear and ill-treatment.[6]

Women often suffer from inequalities in access to education, credit, employment, and divorce. The additional legal inequality they suffer ensures that they have no recourse to the laws against exploitation and abuse, even where these exist. Cultural and religious traditions in parts of the world also make it difficult for women to take their health into their own hands by determining where, when, and with whom they have sexual relations. The claim that women have a right to advice on sexual and reproductive health is an important dimension of the struggle for reproductive rights generally. In addition, violence against women continues to fuel HIV transmission by deterring them from seeking HIV services, or disclosing their status to their partners. In these various ways, the non-observance of human rights becomes in itself a driver of the HIV pandemic.

Stigma, discrimination, and rights

In 2001, in a meeting in Nairobi under the auspices of the World Council of Churches (WCC), African church leaders stated, "the most powerful contribution we can make to combat HIV transmission is the eradication of stigma and discrimination."[7] At the time, child mortality was on the increase, as were the number of children orphaned. Life expectancy was dropping. Health services were stretched to breaking point. National and household reserves and resources were depleted. But most telling was the listing of the many factors contributing to the spread of HIV – among others, the poverty that obstructed efforts to respond to HIV, the fact that the world was no closer to a cure or a vaccine, the many socio-cultural taboos that sabotaged educational efforts by making the discussion of sex and sexuality impossible, and religious and social attitudes that contributed to social stigma.

The Nairobi statement was preceded by an earlier response to HIV and AIDS. In January 2001, representatives of churches, Christian organizations, and their global partners met in Kampala, Uganda. The church, they acknowledged, had been in denial about its own vulnerability to HIV and AIDS. The virus, they realized, spared no one. Courageously, they named cultural practices and perceptions that expose women in particular to the risk of HIV infection, and which were contributing to the steady rise in HIV prevalence. The church, they recognized, "is uniquely placed to combat HIV/AIDS at all levels from the individual to the global and to protect the marginalized and most vulnerable in society." They observed that "the effectiveness of community based initiatives, as well as church involvement in the national commitment to mitigate the impact of HIV and AIDS."[8]

Reading this declaration 15 years later, what strikes me is that these church leaders clearly understood the many barriers that would and could impede their responses. They noted:

> inadequate knowledge, the lack of a clear and common policy direction on prevention, care and support, the reluctance of some of our leaders to share their personal experience of HIV/AIDS to stimulate national conscience, and the persistent culture of silence that has promoted the AIDS stigma and inhibited effective responses in prevention, care and support. We noted the failure of many of our churches to commit local financial and human resources to HIV/AIDS related activities. We recognized the need to encourage, support and involve people living with HIV/AIDS.[9]

These responses were built on the foundation of an earlier WCC statement in 1986, which called for "the right to medical and pastoral care regardless of socio-economic status, race, sex, sexual orientation or sexual relationships" and highlighted an ecumenical consultation's call "to ensure the protection of the human rights of persons affected directly or indirectly by AIDS."[10]

As Sally Smith mentioned in her chapter, during a summit in 2010, religious leaders signed a personal commitment to do more to overcome HIV-related stigma and discrimination. The commitment has since been signed by over 400 religious leaders. In 2013, I researched and wrote a report for the

Ecumenical Advocacy Alliance (EAA), *Together We Must Still Do More: Second Round of Reporting on the Fulfillment of the Personal Commitment to Action on HIV.*[11] The first round of reporting in 2011[12] provided a snapshot of activities and impact the personal commitment had had on the religious leaders who signed. The second round highlighted that cultural and systemic barriers related to the stigma people living with HIV encounter daily still exist, but that the religious leaders themselves had deep personal commitment to respond to HIV to the best of their ability.

Religious leaders have tremendous agency. They have the moral authority to play a major role in determining the directions taken by their communities. They are considered to be role models. Their actions are regarded highly. People believe what they say. They can encourage growth, learning, and action in religious thought, belief, and practice, and they can promote good health and the wellbeing of people in their individual lives, families, local communities, nations, and in the global community.

In the broadest sense, therefore, they have a catalytic function in addressing stigma, denial, and discrimination within communities. The Rev. Canon Gideon Byamugisha is an Anglican priest in Uganda. In 1992, he took the courageous step of disclosing, publicly, the fact that he was living with HIV. Seven years on, this is what he said:

> Stigma has been central to my ministry. You see, where AIDS care and treatment are concerned I'm not a doctor. For scientific research for prevention I'm not a scientist. Where my ministry lies is to work for the defeat of HIV and AIDS-related stigma, shame, denial, discrimination, inaction, and misaction. Millions of people who are HIV positive are not understood. We are not valued and not appreciated. We are dismissed as moral deficits. And that doesn't stop with us as individuals with HIV. The stigma also attaches itself to our families, to our communities, and then it attaches itself to our nations and our continents. . . . Sometimes I will be asked, "You have told us you are HIV positive. Have you ever repented about it?" That's a stigma, [to] connect my infection with immorality. . . . These are stigmatizing instances.[13]

Many people may still find it difficult to see how human rights, considered inherent in all people, can play out in the context of faith. As someone who has lost loved ones to the disease, written about it, and worked in global AIDS advocacy for many years, I know without any doubt that stigma can be a wall that allows no one over or through it. I know, too, that a stigmatizing community is a divided community that is, in itself, in need of healing. Stigma divides families and communities. It is a barrier to effective health care. In the broadest sense, it is incompatible with health itself. Stigma is a health-care issue because it is designed to bar people, deemed somehow unworthy of society's respect and compassion from accessing the life-enhancing services and support they so urgently need.

So in order to respond to HIV, you don't have to be a doctor or a nurse. You don't have to run hospitals or clinics or voluntary counseling or homecare programs, although all of those are excellent ways that religiously motivated groups are currently contributing to the response to HIV. It was Archbishop Desmond Tutu who said, "Your ordinary acts of love and hope point to the extraordinary promise that every human life is of inestimable value."[14] And that is a contribution every one of us can make to the healthcare agenda that will, eventually, stop the advance of HIV.

Resources

Now More than Ever (available in EN, FR, RU, ESP and German). http://www.hivhumanrightsnow.org/10-reasons/.

Stories of Hope: Experiences of Pregnant Women and Mothers Living with HIV. http://www.icaso.org/media/files/23935-StoriesofStigmaStoriesofHopeENno-DateSpreadsWebReady.pdf

Together We Must Still Do More: Second Round of Reporting on the Fulfillment of the Personal Commitment to Action on HIV. Available through EAA.

Questions for discussion

• Do people with HIV or AIDS have the same rights as others to health care and treatment? Do they have fewer rights? Do they have more rights?

• Supposing that healthcare facilities for people with HIV or AIDS are available where you live, what might deter you from seeking help or advice from them?

Part Two

Contextual Struggles

AIDS comes to break the bonds so present in religious communities: those of misinformation on the subject and the lack of understanding of sexuality as God's gift. It is a fact that the reality of AIDS makes us question our certainties.
– Ester Lisboa, Brazil

Discrimination on any basis, be it caste, race, creed, color, gender, sexual orientation, HIV or any other medical condition, disability etc amounts to rejection of the Trinitarian God of life.
– Metropolitan Dr Geevarghese Coorilos, India

If we can agree on nothing else today except that to continue to demonize drug users is not the way forward, then we have achieved something.
– Mags Maher, United Kingdom

I have been with people who have been mired in the very same dark holes of self-hatred because of what their families and faith communities have made them believe all this while. I have seen that all of them have come to find

an affirmation that God loves them and there is nothing
at all to fix because we were never broken to begin with.
– "Marcus"

In Part Two of this publication, we invited some dozen or so individuals to put flesh on the themes explored in Part One by reflecting on the issue of human rights and HIV from the standpoint of their own experience. Each of our contributors has been personally affected by HIV or AIDS, professionally or in their own bodies or families, their churches or their friendship groups. It has taken courage to write in this way: and yet the big issues we discussed in Part One come alive only when we read them against the lives of women, men, and children in their contexts and their communities.

Some of the experiences individuals have had with faith communities have been highly negative, some opinions and suggested responses may be very controversial. These should be understood as personal stories and reflections. We are immensely grateful for the courage and honesty of our writers. We have testimonies, throughout this book, of the silence that often surrounds the epidemic. Breaking that silence is never easy.

Chapter 6

Reflecting on the Role of Networks of People Living with HIV

JP Mokgethi-Heath

Networks for people living with HIV (PLHIV) started essentially as support groups. In the 1980s, when no medication was available to treat HIV, the networks provided space for people to meet and discuss what they were going through. And much of what people were going through was related to the stigma and discrimination experience by PLHIV. Particularly in Europe and North America, the vast majority of PLHIV were gay men who, in addition to the stigma and discrimination they experienced related to HIV, also were alienated by their faith communities because of their sexual orientation. By 1986, the Global Network of People living with HIV (GNP+) was founded, followed by the foundation of the International AIDS Society (IAS) in 1988. Only in 1992 was the International Community of Women living with HIV (ICW) founded: in those early days it was incorrectly believed that HIV was primarily a problem for men. Strong advocacy for the rights of PLHIV had started. The voice that now echoes from many people on the margins – "Nothing for us without us" – originated within networks of PLHIV. During the 1994 Paris AIDS Summit, 42 countries committed to the GIPA Principle – Greater Involvement of People living with AIDS in the decision-making processes that affects their lives.

The path of standing up for their rights forced these networks of PLHIV to a clear Human Rights focus, including rights to equality in work, education, protection under the law, the right to medication and treatment, and above all a life of dignity regardless of their HIV status. While statements about HIV from a faith perspective had already been made by the World Council of Churches (WCC) as early as 1986, it was not until 2002, when the African Network of Religious Leaders living with or personally affected by HIV (ANERELA+) was formed, that there was an overtly faith-based network of PLHIV. In a much more concrete way, this challenged the stigmatizing messages of judgment and exclusion that continued to flow from religious communities. By 2003, GNP+ was already committed to finding clearer ways of working in faith-related issues, and chose to host the official launch of ANERELA+ in Kampala in October of that year.

This close collaboration between the different PLHIV networks has meant a cross-pollination of ideas and capacities. Faith related networks have learned about human rights and more secular networks have learned about faith and the importance of it in the lives of many PLHIV. Today the journey made by PLHIV networks has inspired the voices of many other people living on the fringes of human rights to raise their own voices with the cry: "Nothing for us without us."

Phumzile Mabizela

The People Living with HIV (PLHIV) movement is not as strong as it was about five years ago.[1] Most funders have changed their focus, even as some countries still experience new infections every day. Living with HIV, I have learned that human rights are universal; but they go hand-in-hand with responsibilities. Over the years, the PLHIV movement has kept track of progress made to end AIDS. Today, one of the challenges the movement is responding to is to make sure that all people living with HIV have access to crucial services like regular monitoring tests of viral load and CD4 count. I have had access to medication and other services as a result of the advocacy that has been done by all sectors. This is sound public health strategy, because early access to medication for all people living with HIV will significantly reduce the numbers of new infections. My concern is that pharmaceutical companies are still making it difficult for poor countries to have the right to produce their own medication. Their main focus is on profit and not on saving lives.

For me the PLHIV movement is both a pastoral movement and an advocacy one. Both are important: the pastoral focus, because people are dying due to lack of resources and support; the advocacy focus, in order to hold the decision-makers accountable and to keep challenging the rich countries to make resources available for research until a cure is found.

While secular human rights voices have done an excellent job, we would not be where we are today without the ecumenical faith-based movement. Faith-based voices stress that we are all created in the image of God regardless of our race, class, gender, sexual orientation, or political beliefs. Most hospitals in Africa are run by faith-based organizations, while smaller centres have made sure that people have access to care, medication, and support. Because nutrition is so important, some faith-based organizations have focused on food sovereignty, ensuring that communities can make decisions on the production and distribution of food.

But the whole movement is more than just an African movement. It is bigger and more connected. We have a number of common challenges whether we are in Africa or in other parts of the world, and our unity has made our voices stronger. But I am deeply concerned that funding for HIV has shrunk dramatically, and this is where religious voices could help. For example, countries like Thailand and the Philippines have a growing epidemic, but the religious leaders who are living with HIV are reluctant to disclose their status or live openly and positively as agents of change. Societal resistance is often based on the stigma and discrimination associated with sexual orientation and the inclusion of sexual minorities. It is a slow process, but the more people are exposed to accurate information on sexuality, the more their attitudes towards LGBTI communities can and will change.

I am an African woman religious leader, living with HIV, who is in a leadership position. This has given other women hope that they can become leaders even after diagnosis. Most religious leaders are male, so it has been important to lead the recognition of the challenges faced by women who are living with HIV. These challenges include issues of sexual and reproductive health and rights, which make women and girls in Africa so vulnerable to HIV. Antiretrovirals for instance have different side effects for different genders. Gender inequality has also made it difficult for women to negotiate safer sex. The development of women-controlled prevention methods should be a priority, but it does not seem to be high on the list for researchers.

Thinking forward, the PLHIV movement has to make sure that the voices of representatives from "key populations" of particularly vulnerable people are heard, so that those who are most vulnerable to HIV do not become invisible. We must make sure that HIV and AIDS remains in the UN's Sustainable Development Goals for as long as possible. Most countries only have access to a limited number of ARV regimens and this has to change. More positive theologies on sexuality have to be developed. If we want future generations to have a more positive attitude towards sex and sexuality, our teachings on sex have to change drastically. And sexual and reproductive health and rights must be discussed within spaces of worship. It is a matter of life and death.

Chapter 7

Evidence and Experience
of Key Populations

Sex Work, Human Rights and the Church
Peninah Mwangi

Sex work is the provision of sexual services for money or goods. A sex worker is a sister, a cousin, an aunt, and a mother to members of your community. She is a member of your community!

Religious leaders find it difficult to have open communication about human sexuality. Even though most religions affirm sex as a good gift of God, sexuality still seems like a threatening taboo topic, only to be discussed in vague terms. Sex work takes it further.

The women who sell sex the world over are subjected to repressive and discriminatory laws and practices which in turn fuel stigma, discrimination, and in a large number of instances violence being perpetrated against sex workers.

In 2007, BHESP, a sex worker organization in Kenya, applied for funding from a Christian organization for HIV prevention. The response was clear: "We cannot fund sex workers to continue to remain in a disempowered situation."

Female sex workers are 13.5 times more likely than females in the general population to be infected with HIV. With heightened risks of HIV and other sexually transmitted infections, sex workers face substantial barriers in accessing prevention, treatment, and care services, largely because of stigma, discrimination, and criminalization in the societies in which they live. These social, legal, and economic injustices contribute to their high risk – and, by extension, the general population – of acquiring HIV.

A study carried out by BHESP in Thika town (Kenya) shows that 80 percent of sex workers are Christians. Sixty percent of sex workers in Thika attend church regularly, and 20 percent tithe. Eighty percent of sex workers with children have had them baptized in church. Let me share some of their quotes with you:

> *"Members of our small Christian community refused to hold prayers in my house because I am a sex worker."* – Flora

(In the Kenyan Christian community, much importance is attached to small Christian community members meeting in one's house for prayers.)

> *"When our colleague who was also a sex worker died, we hired a man of God to lead her burial because her pastor had refused."* – Njeri

> *"When I started to work as a sex worker, I had to stop going to my church because the members said I had fallen and some could not sit next to me."* – Agness

Our experience shows that HIV and AIDS prevention is particularly difficult because of the stigma associated with the disease. Religious teachings and practices have intensified this stigma by "labelling" persons infected as "sinners" and treating persons as second- or even third-class citizens. Key populations (in other words, transgender individuals, men who have sex with men, sex workers, and people who use drugs) have suffered the brunt of these stigmatizing practices. According to a sex worker in Thika, "My pastor refused to baptize my daughter because I could not present the father, but had been taking my contributions to church without asking how I earned the money."

I have observed that sex work in Africa is generally viewed through a lens of morality. Instead of embracing everyone as sister and brother, the tendency is to categorize and judge others as less worthy and outside the realm of religion. By focusing on religious doctrines and ethical teachings, too often religious leaders either cannot see or are unwilling to recognize the realities of human behaviour. In my church, our priest adheres to moral principles deemed divine during his sermons regardless of human consequences. In most cases he is more eager to preserve the "purity" or "correctness" of the church's theological perspective than to protect human lives. My church opposes condoms because it is against artificial birth control and believes that their promotion encourages promiscuity.

"Some of my clients are the highest contributors in Church, and they are always asked to greet the congregation from the pulpit" – Nelly

"The church preaches against use of condoms; I would rather leave church but be able to live to feed my children." – Mercy

Religious beliefs, attitudes, teachings, and practices can contribute both negative and positive dimensions to efforts aimed at promoting HIV and AIDS prevention. Some religious leaders and faith-based communities are taking a positive, pro-active role in the struggle against HIV and AIDS, albeit with an attitude toward key populations that can only be described as moralistic. In Kenya, the teachings of most religious groups stress care and compassion, love and life, hope and healing. They affirm the worth and dignity of every human being and that every person is made in the image of God and is to be cherished, protected, and preserved. The general perception of the population (including the laws that are made) is influenced by the religious leaders.

Yet, without addressing the human rights violations perpetrated on key populations, merely providing HIV prevention and treatment services will remain an insufficient and misguided response. Based on our experience, we recommend that HIV responses for key populations ensure their human rights through active promotion of equality and non-discrimination in accessing prevention and interventions across the full continuum of care. By focusing on the human rights of every person including key populations, religious groups can become partners and champions in fighting stigma and discrimination and hence influence the general population.

Stigma against key populations can be overcome if the highest values of the faith are stressed: namely, love and compassion, hope and health.

My Role as an Advocate for the International Network of People Who Use Drugs (INPUD)
Mags Maher

> HIV is a greater threat to the public and individual health than drug misuse. (ACMD, 1988)

I am here today as part of a movement of drug user activists who are fighting for the rights to life, sexual, and reproductive health, change, acknowledgement, and acceptance in society without prejudice or marginalization. I have 25 years of experience working in the drug and alcohol field. I started to use drugs at the age of 13 to alleviate the pain of incest-related abuse. During these last 35 years I have relapsed three times, reverting to problematic drug use. At one point in my life I was termed "a multiple crack injector" and would inject up to 20 times a day.

Throughout my life I have come into contact and belonged to Christian churches, including the Pentecostal Church, the Catholic Church, the Reformed Evangelical Church, and a Baptist Church with Calvinist teachings, the Baptist Free Church, the Brethren, and Jehovah's Witnesses. The common thread amongst all these denominations was that as soon as I mentioned that I was an active drug user, I was told to stop using drugs. I was told that if I was "a true believer then this would not be a problem." Otherwise I should step down from the church's membership or be excommunicated, as I was backslider. I was denied partaking in holy communion, and told that I did not truly have salvation and that if I expected to remain an active member of the church I was expected to stop using drugs. The reasons I was given for this would vary. They included: I was desecrating the temple of God (my physical body); I was not walking in the likeness of God; or I was actively sinning every day and therefore could not truly be saved – the list goes on.

In the end, wanting to know the purpose/existence of humans, and due to my interest in original sin, I enrolled in Bible School to study theology and find some of the answers for myself. What I left with was a personal understanding that "God so loved the whole world that he gave his only begotten Son to die on the cross" for sinners like you and me. More importantly, I gained an understanding of original sin that is not based on what is right or wrong but is determined by the conviction that we feel in our hearts every time we go against what God has laid down as the best path for us on which to live our lives. With Christ's righteousness put into our hearts, once we receive salvation we are given his strength to try and become more like him. But just because we become "Christians" it does not mean that we suddenly stop sinning, because, as the apostle Paul so rightly points out in Romans 7, "For I do not do what I want, but I do the very thing that I hate." Sin lives within us all and creation groans in anticipation of the return of our Lord Jesus Christ.

In the eyes of the church and society, drug users are generally often seen as a scourge; a marginalized group without a voice living on the very fringes of society. Many drug users, even if they have a faith and belief in God, find they are unable to approach their church leaders and disclose their drug use out of fear of further judgment, discrimination, and marginalization.

As drug users, we don't advocate for an immoral world. We are not anti-community. In fact, some of my deepest experiences of belonging and love have been with my peers within the drug-using community. Yet when we are pushed to the fringes of society and we are not believed but instead criminalized, it reduces our chances of accessing treatment.

Father Carmelo, who is known by many still today in the East End of London, was a lovely gentle man, a bit of an unorthodox Catholic priest who dedicated his life to serving the Italian community in and around Mile End. In the late 1990s, he formed a team of peer advocates from the community, all of whom who were active drug users, to provide terminal care for more than 60 of our peers who were dying from AIDS-related complications. During this time I experienced some of the deepest acts of love and compassion. Our friends were able to die with dignity and respect. At the same time in the Netherlands, a Lutheran priest ran a drug consumption room for drug users so that they would be able to walk into a clean, clinical room and inject their drugs safely without fear of recriminations or judgments. There have also been examples in America of some churches running needle exchanges and ensuring that clean drug paraphernalia are distributed to people who inject drugs in their community.

While many faith-based groups still reject drug users, the examples that I have given of the work of the church in grassroots communities show what a huge difference it can make if judgmental, self-righteous attitudes can be changed in favour of providing access to support, opportunities, health care, and most importantly prevention and risk reduction of HIV. And abstinence is not a solution.

Harm reduction is literally a life or death situation for many of my peers. It has become a vehicle for solidarity and respect, and harm reduction practice itself saves lives and enables drug users to have access to a language that helps them speak openly, in a positive and empowering way about their drug use. We need to adopt a harm-reduction approach, as it improves communication between diverse groups, it is useful in evaluating the effectiveness of interventions and policies, it maps out the territory and identifies gaps, and in short, it helps us stop making things up as we go along. It is a pragmatic approach that is based on prioritizing goals, has humanist values, focuses on risks and harm, does not focus on abstinence, and seeks to maximize the range of intervention options that are available. Harm reduction has allowed drug users to start owning their experiences and sharing them with others, and using their experiences to illustrate and promote positive change. By reducing the stigma associated with drug use, in many ways all those seemingly meaningless experiences from the past are suddenly meaningful.

IDU and HIV Transmission

Injection drug use is the main method of HIV transmission in Central and Eastern Europe.

Drug use is widespread.

The United Nations Office for Drug Control and Crime Prevention estimates that worldwide, 185 million people each year consumed illicit drugs from 1998-2000.

United Nations Office for Drug Control and Crime Prevention.

– Global Illicit Drug Trends 2002. New York: UNODCCP.

INPUD's aim is to build capacity at a global level to be able to speak about HIV, and to build peer involvement on a global stage to address the complexities and challenges of being a drug user. If we can agree on nothing else today except that to continue to demonize drug users is not the way forward, then we have achieved something. Finding out why people want to use drugs in the first place is far more productive and will allow for an honest debate, as well as allow us to live in a less repressive society. Mutual aid, peer support and community strategies are all areas that INPUD has enormous knowledge about and that it could use to support churches. Current punitive drug policies and the war on drugs cost a fortune. They do not save lives; all they are good for is bad policy decision making that ultimately leads to our community dying – and, most certainly, you cannot rehabilitate anyone once they are dead. The only logical way forward is to decriminalize drug use and bring back the voice of the drug user.

Sexuality and Self-Worth

Marcus

I was sitting in front of my HIV doctor when he asked what my job is. I told him I am a nurse. "How come you are HIV positive? You should have known better," he said.

I felt small.

"I know Doc but it is more complicated than that," I replied.

He handed me my script for my supply of ARVs and called another patient inside, and I left that room and passed through a long queue of guys waiting for their turn. I felt nothing more than just a hospital code.

I have told myself a million times that "I should have known better" since I tested reactive for HIV. I have been through four years of university and did countless sessions of health education on safer sex and universal precautions. Why did I not protect myself?

I have to confess, I never really thought of myself as even worth protecting.

My mother raised me and my brother alone as my father raised another family. As a school teacher, she had no choice but to leave us with relatives while she had to work. I was left with cousins and uncles.

I was sexually abused, and I was five.

I didn't realize it was even abuse until later. I was an overachieving and devout Catholic schoolboy, as some achievements gave me some affirmation that I was good. But I grew up aloof and confused by feelings and dreams I started to feel ashamed about. I had no one to talk to. I prayed so hard for the dreams to stop.

I was 11 and went to one of our regular confessions. I confessed that I started to have sexual thoughts about some of my classmates. I was in an all-boys school. The priest stood up and pointed his finger at me and shouted that I was going to hell.

I have always considered God as my father. He protected me from my nightmares. But then God hated me. I would pretend to be sick to go to the infirmary when it was time for catechism class on the ten commandments. All that staring made me sick.

I was 14 when I first sold sex. I was walking home and a car stopped by. It was quick cash and God hated me anyway.

Also by that time I found a way to numb myself with alcohol and discovered that I can fly away with different substances.

I lived a double life. I got myself through nursing school through a scholarship. I did everything to make myself feel that I am less broken.

This other hidden life was a window into how it is for people who are driven to live underground because of what society dictates is morally upright. In the closet, where no one can judge us, we find others, seeking for some affirmation that we are worth some warmth and compassion. No matter how temporary, some are willing to even pay cash for it.

I have always known the unsafe world I got myself into. I went to HIV clinics to get tested but then never came back for the result. It was only when one of my friends got AIDS that I finally confirmed that I am HIV positive.

Testing HIV positive for me seemed to be God's punishment for my lifestyle. He hates me for who I am. I am worthy of a disease.

I have never been so creative in planning ways to kill myself. When I had an adverse reaction from Nevirapine during my ARV trial, I wished the high fever would finally kill me. When I tried to regain some hope about life, I applied for an international scholarship. I declared my HIV status and thought that it would be an advantage, as they stated preferential option for people with disabilities. They rejected my application. Maybe it was my new drug, Efavirenz, but for me HIV killed my dreams, and I wished that I had thrown myself in front of a truck.

It was a dead end for me then. That is until I found a faith-based support group for people living with HIV in the Philippines. With every seeker I met at the meetings, I found someone who shared the same wounds of being pushed to the margins because of who they are. I have been with people who have been mired in the very same dark holes of self-hatred because of what their families and faith communities have made them believe all this while. I have seen that all of them have come to find an affirmation that God loves them and there is nothing at all to fix, for we were never broken to begin with.

We all support each other with deep prayer and sincere presence and friendship. I have felt God's love flowing through each of us in providing support for each other and doing everything right for our wellness while living with HIV.

My scars will always be there to remind me of what wrong can be made right. From where I have come from to where I am now, I believe that sexuality is part of creation that God deems good. It is a gift for all humanity for creating relationships and mutual love. Issues on gender, sex, and sexuality continue to be a hard struggle within the predominantly Roman Catholic Filipino society.

Today, I am grateful that I am surrounded by people who affirm that my experiences, gifts, and graces are essential tools in our HIV prevention work, and who affirm that sex and the diversity of gender and sexuality are gifts from God. Along with our faith communities and the PLHIV community, I live and work toward that day that no one will ever be condemned and excluded simply for being who they truly are.

Questions for Discussion

- In your church or community, can you or others talk honestly and openly to one another about social concerns that may include sex work, people using drugs, men who have sex with men? If not, what could be done differently that would allow safe and open discussion?

- Open and honest discussion does not mean everyone in the end will agree on what is right or wrong. So what would you hope such discussion might achieve?

- How may our judgment of and discrimination against people who use drugs, engage in sex work, are transgender, or have same-sex relationships, lead to them being pushed further to the edges of society? How may compassion make a difference in your and their lives?

Chapter 8

Just Care and the Image of God: An Orthodox Perspective on HIV, AIDS, and Human Rights

Geevarghese Coorilos

The central Orthodox theological paradigms of the holy Trinity and trinitarian life are of huge significance in addressing issues of human rights, dignity, freedom, and grace. Life is essentially a theological principle and an ethical postulate. All life, without any distinction whatsoever, is a sacred gift of the triune God. What characterizes life within the community of the holy Trinity are justice, dignity, mutuality, sharing, and interdependence. The dignity and equality of each person in the triune community are affirmed. Therefore, discrimination on any basis – be it caste, race, creed, colour, gender, sexual orientation, HIV, or any other medical condition or disability – amounts to rejection of the trinitarian God of life.

The holy Trinity presupposes values of care, justice, mutuality, and grace. HIV and AIDS call for an ethic of care from a human rights/justice perspective. What is distinctly Christian about our attitude toward people affected by HIV and AIDS is the compassionate and caring outlook that Jesus exemplified in his life and ministry. I prefer to call this approach, an ethic of "just care," which is a trinitarian formula and therefore a communitarian model of care, itself modeled after a communitarian/trinitarian God. Within the holy Trinity, the Father, Son and the Holy Spirit cohere among one another. Whatever happens within the family affects everyone else at all levels.

In the context of HIV and AIDS, a trinitarian model of just care would imply that when there is a person who is affected by HIV or AIDS, everyone in the community shares the pain and suffering of the affected person. As the trinitarian God of life is one who suffers with others, a fellow sufferer, we are called to identify ourselves with those in pain and suffering. In this sense, an ethic of just care is about embracing the issue of HIV and AIDS and also about embracing people with HIV and AIDS. When we accept the challenge of caring for people with HIV and AIDS, we are in fact sharing in the common Humanity, Identity, and Vulnerability (sharing in HIV) of all human beings.

Orthodox ethics tend to avoid discourses that are moralistic in nature and content. Moralism does not solve the issue of HIV and AIDS. Instead it stands in the way of providing care to the needy. Rather than putting the blame on certain sections of people (e.g., sexual minorities), an ethic of just care addresses socio-economic and political structures – such as capitalism, patriarchy, racism, and Caste-ism – that cause and spread the disease. In this sense, a just care ethic goes beyond a charity approach toward those affected by HIV and AIDS and addresses the concern as a political challenge of defending dignity and rights as human beings.

The "image of God," another key principle in Orthodox theological anthropology, particularly in Patristic theology, is perhaps one of the most fundamental moral imperatives for human rights advocacy and action. The affirmation that humanity has been created in God's image and likeness implies that every human being is equal and that violations of human rights and dignity would therefore amount to distortion of the divine image in humanity. This message echoed powerfully in my ears during a meeting when an HIV affected mother narrated her story of alienation and discrimination from her own kith and kin and when she urged us: "My dear sisters and brothers, I would like you to know that I have only lost some measure of my immunity, not my humanity. I am still a human being, so treat me as one."

Question for discussion

- The writer suggests that Orthodox ethics tend to avoid discourses that are moralistic in nature and content. In relation to HIV and AIDS, what difference would it make to our understanding of human rights if we followed that example?

Chapter 9

Theological Challenges and Opportunities in Addressing Human Rights, Sexuality, and HIV: An African Perspective

Ezra Chitando

Some African political leaders, such as Robert Mugabe of Zimbabwe, have asserted that the very concept of human rights is part of the larger enterprise of colonialism. Along with some African intellectuals, they maintain that the idea of human rights emerges from the global North's unfair engagement with the global South. They lampoon the call for human rights, charging that the same countries that clamour for human rights have been responsible for some of the most appalling crimes against humanity. Mugabe and his school of African intellectuals quickly retrieve the memory of slavery, colonialism, and the skewed global economic system to justify their contention. The rhetorical power of their argument can be seen in how popular Mugabe is in the global South. He is presented as the Suffering Servant who is sacrificed for standing up for the rights of the Africans against the principalities and powers of this world.

To examine the theological challenges and opportunities in addressing human rights and issues that come with HIV, such as sexuality, in the African context, requires that we look at a number of issues: the politicization of human rights; the challenges that emerge from addressing human rights and HIV, with particular reference to sexuality; and the opportunities that are available in responding to this theme.

"We died for these human rights": An overview of the contestation over human rights

The discourse on human rights has elicited an ultra-defensive stance among some African (and other global South) politicians and intellectuals. Whereas the call for the human rights of marginalized groups such as sex workers, men who have sex with men, injecting drug users, and others has come to the fore in the context of addressing HIV, some African politicians and intellectuals have argued that the emphasis on human rights is a Western ploy to dominate Africa. They seek to marshal a number of arguments to defend their stance. In this section, I seek to uphold a descriptive approach. Although I do not subscribe to these arguments, it is critical to appreciate how they are constructed, as well as to understand why they appeal to many people.

First, building their case on the foundation of cultural relativism, some critics maintain that there are underlying and fundamental differences in culture in the global North and in the global South. One of the persistent arguments is that whereas in the global North individualism dominates, communalism dominates in the global South. They argue that in those contexts where the good of the community receives emphasis ahead of individual interests, references to human rights must contend with the rights of the larger community. Thus, individual persons must be understood within the context of their location in community. Consequently, they conclude, there is need to acknowledge that approaches to human rights will differ in the global South.

A second argument refers to the emotional/historical dimension of human rights. As outlined in the introduction, some African politicians such as Mugabe appeal to emotions to question the call for human rights in Africa. Rhetorically, Mugabe has asked, "Where was the West when we died for these human rights?" This tactic is quite powerful as it introduces a hermeneutic of suspicion and seeks to remind African activists of their continent's history. It evokes the memory of oppression and exclusion to persuade Africans to be wary of joining the call for universal human rights. Other African intellectuals move in to buttress this point by claiming that the whole discourse on human rights perpetuates the colonial stereotype. Africa (and the global South) is portrayed as a savage and backward continent that needs to be lectured on human rights in order to ensure that "light" comes to the "dark continent."

Third, it is argued that human rights are deployed as a smokescreen to effect regime change in Africa. Once again, this argument is articulated with force and persuasion by political leaders such as Mugabe. They strongly contend that predominantly Western governments have used the "abuse of human rights" argument to remove governments that do not share their agenda. The typical argument uses the proverbial saying that when a leopard wants to eat its little ones, it first accuses them of smelling like a goat. According to this line of thinking, governments that resist Western powers are accused of oppressing their citizens and posing a threat to global stability. Their countries are then invaded, the leaders are deposed, and the West shares the spoils. As with the emotional/historical dimension to human rights, this argument appeals to some people; Saddam Hussein in Iraq and Muammar Gaddafi in Libya are examples of this trend.

Fourth is the tendency to evoke religious and cultural values as overriding (some) human rights. The major contention is that human rights are built on a secular approach to life. This approach comes under fire when critics charge that most of the people in the global South are guided by a religious approach to life. They further argue that religious and cultural values must not be subordinated to human rights. Essentially, this approach senses a fundamental clash between human rights on the one hand and religious/cultural values on the other.

Human sexuality and HIV: Challenges

The arguments outlined above have been prominent in responses to HIV in the global South. In particular, the theme of human sexuality has generated many challenges. While it is accepted that sexual transmission accounts for most HIV cases, there has been contestation over prevention methods. The religious and cultural argument has tended to frustrate efforts to address human sexuality in the era of HIV. Those who uphold conservative views have insisted that there are key religious and cultural values (such as the sacredness of sex, for example) that should not be tampered with, even in the face of the crisis.

Conservative interpreters of African traditional, Christian, and Muslim traditions and scriptures have been adamant that there are "timeless" values relating to sex and sexuality that must be upheld. As a result, they have resisted comprehensive sexuality education and information for children and youth. They (wrongly) conclude that equipping children and youth with knowledge, information, and skills relating to human sexuality will promote experimentation and de-sacralization of sexuality. Such conservative interpretations of religious traditions and sacred texts have emerged as a challenge in responding to HIV.

Emerging directly from such interpretations is the controversy over same-sex relationships. Many African religious leaders have argued that same-sex relationships are against the core teachings of their religions. In particular, leaders from African Traditional Religions, Christianity, and Islam have asserted that references to the rights of homosexuals are not sustainable in the face of the teachings of their specific religions. This has generated considerable controversy, as activists have maintained that such interpretations are faulty.

Although the era of HIV requires open and honest discussions on human sexuality in its complexity and diversity, opponents of the human rights approach have used religious and cultural arguments to frustrate more realistic approaches. They have also challenged the promotion of gender justice, arguing that there is a "divine order" that must be upheld at all times. When there have been calls to uphold the rights of sex workers, for example, they have fiercely opposed such moves. However, alternative approaches exist that can yield better results.

Human sexuality and HIV: Opportunities

The notion that human rights and religious values are locked in mortal combat is fundamentally flawed. There is need for creativity in persuading conservative religious leaders to appreciate the importance of promoting human rights in the era of HIV. First, we must invest in bridging the gap between human rights terminology and theological concepts. The experience of faith-based organizations that have embraced the rights-based approach shows that it is possible to change attitudes when a less confrontational approach is adopted. For instance, the International Network of Religious leaders living with or personally affected by HIV and AIDS (INERELA) and the Ecumenical HIV and AIDS Initiatives and Advocacy (EHAIA) have learned the value of framing human rights concepts in theological understandings. For example, where the Universal Declaration of Human Rights refers to the "inherent dignity and equal and inalienable rights of all members of the human family," the theological understanding that "all human beings are created equal before God" resonates more deeply with religious leaders.

In order to make progress when addressing issues of human sexuality in the era of HIV, it is prudent to couch human rights principles in theological concepts that are appealing to religious leaders. Across the diverse religious traditions, concepts such as love, justice, solidarity and compassion are universally recognized as central to the lives of believers. These beliefs and practices are central to promoting the rights of marginalized groups and individuals. Most religious leaders are willing to tone down conservative positions when human rights are articulated in familiar theological concepts.

While the idea that human rights are a foreign imposition appeals to some people, this can be countered by highlighting indigenous African concepts. For example, the notion of *Ubuntu* (humanness) can be utilized to promote human rights in Africa. Ubuntu contends that one's wellbeing is intrinsically related to the wellbeing of the "other." Essentially, Ubuntu declares, "I am, because you are." This concept can be appealed to when engaging religious leaders and gatekeepers of culture to promote the acceptance of marginalized groups and individuals. What is required is a detailed analysis of the concept and its implications for ensuring that nobody is left behind in the response to HIV.

Other opportunities for promoting human rights within the religious sector in the face of HIV relate to the need to promote re-readings of sacred texts and traditions. EHAIA and INERELA have employed the Contextual Bible Study (CBS) methodology to challenge conservative interpretations of sacred texts and traditions. Through participatory community readings of sacred texts, new and liberating interpretations have emerged. This has facilitated open and honest dialogue around sex and sexuality, diversity, and social justice.

Africa's protracted struggle against colonialism and discrimination is another valuable entry point in promoting human rights. Numerous African politicians and intellectuals recognize that many of the continent's citizens have had to launch armed struggles in the quest for liberation. This memory of resisting oppression can be appealed to when promoting human rights in the face of HIV in Africa. We can then place the struggle for the rights of marginalized groups within the context of the struggle for liberation that the continent has waged.

Conclusion

The debate over human rights has emerged as a major challenge to effective responses to HIV by communities of faith, particularly in Africa. This challenge is unfortunate, given the fact that communities of faith have played a major role in responding to HIV. I have outlined the key arguments that have been used to resist rights-based approaches to HIV in Africa. I have highlighted the insistence of some African politicians and intellectuals that the global North lacks the moral authority to promote human rights to the global South. I have also drawn attention to some of the challenges that have emerged in efforts to address pressing issues such as human sexuality in the era of HIV, summarizing the tendency of some religious leaders to regard human rights and religious values as being oppositional. Opportunities are also available for effective interventions. While some challenges exist in promoting a human rights culture in addressing HIV, I am confident that employing a creative and consultative approach that addresses the fears and concerns of religious leaders will allow us to develop more sustainable responses.

Questions for discussion

- Is "human rights" language appealing or divisive in your culture? What concepts and language from your own culture provide alternatives or parallels to human rights?

- In contexts where human rights are being represented as tools of post-colonial oppression, how should those who wish to defend rights but live outside the country or context speak and act?

Chapter 10

From Apartheid Activism to AIDS Advocacy: A South African Perspective

Callie Long

It was the late 1980s.[1] Those engaged in the often-deadly resistance against apartheid were witnessing the violent but dying struggles of a regime that had over four decades systematically stripped people of their dignity and human rights through forced legislation. Reductive and inhumane, the pariah state was crumbling under the gaze of a world that recoiled in revulsion from the naked racism of apartheid South Africa, as it had from the horrors of the Holocaust, naming it as one of the biggest moral problems of a post–World War II reality.

"The global imagination was deeply offended, and felt that something must be done," explained Professor Jim Cochrane in an interview in September 2014. Professor Cochrane, a South African, holds the positions of Emeritus Professor of Religious Studies and Senior Research Associate in the School of Public Health and Family Medicine at the University of Cape Town, and is also an Adjunct Professor in the Department of Social Sciences and Health Policy of the Wake Forest School of Medicine in the US. He has spent much of his academic career researching and writing about religion and public health, public life, and globalization, including studying and documenting South Africa's history within the context of theology and politics and their wide-ranging impact on the country's course from a dark past to liberation, and from repression to freedom.

Taking the discussion back to the early days of colonization, Cochrane spoke about its legacy, as well as the significance of the theatre of war – both global and regional – on the history of activism in South Africa. The rise and eventual demise of Afrikaner nationalism, parallel to the rise of African liberation movements – such as the African National Congress, the Black Consciousness Movement, and the United Democratic Front, supported by international allies – were also momentous. In this, he highlighted the colossal impact of the great thinkers and human rights activists of the time – people like Steve Biko, Robert Sobukwe, Mahatma Ghandi, Julius Nyerere, Oliver Thambo, Beyers Naudé, Mahmood Mamdani, Martin Luther King, and Martin Niemöller – on the anti-apartheid struggle and its discourse about "what it means to be human." Bolstered by the support of such institutions and organizations as the UN, the International Labour Organization, the World Council of Churches, and locally, the South African Council of Churches and the Christian Institute of South Africa, the liberation movement gained strength. It was deeply interwoven in the radical critique of apartheid and a general "ethic of paternalism applied to Africans" by white society that shaped power relations was the language of human rights; as Cochrane explained, "Racism, like sexism or slavery, rests on a view of the other as a 'minor' who cannot be given the full rights of an adult."

"The question of human rights was critical to this discourse, as are the fundamental moral responsibilities that come with the spiritual capacity of being human," Cochrane noted:

> As far as we can tell, human beings are unique in this regard. Not only do we delight in creation itself, but we possess the capacity to imagine what does not exist in nature with the ability to bring it into being. This not only enables us to change things, but also to destroy things. So it carries a moral responsibility. Every time we do something, we face that question: for what reason, for whose good, for what intent, for what purpose? These are fundamental moral questions. It is I think [also] the religious question.

A new enemy

The 1980s and the early 1990s were a time of political and social upheaval in South Africa. However, the current had shifted, and in 1994, on April 27, millions of South Africans lined up over three days to participate in the general election; the first in which all adult citizens could take part and one that would see Nelson Mandela installed as the country's first democratically elected President.

The decades-long resistance that pre-dates the Universal Declaration on Human Rights (1948) and the later African Charter on Human and People's Rights, go back to the 1800s into the 20th Century, and can in part trace its roots to the anti-slavery and labour movements. Yet, even as this struggle culminated in the historic celebration of universal suffrage, a deadly spectre hovered. A disease, identified as the human immunodeficiency virus (HIV), was wreaking havoc with humans' immune systems worldwide. In the early days, it claimed the lives of hundreds of people daily, leaving few unaffected. South Africa was not spared. It was a disease of epidemic proportions that attracted cultural and normative precepts steeped in moral judgment, and would become a lightning rod for stigma and biases. As apartheid had dominated cultural and political conversation for so long, the dominant narrative now would focus on HIV and its attendant acquired immune deficiency syndrome (AIDS).

For those engaged in anti-apartheid civil action, there were strong touch points between the activism related to human rights and that to HIV. "Thanks to the powerful actors that emerged in the anti-apartheid struggle, South Africa has a strong history of civil society action, and many committed, passionate people, some of whom acquired HIV, now took on this new fight," said Cochrane. They would be pitted against a disease that was often a battle of life and death before the advent of antiretroviral treatment. It was a new struggle, and one that would ultimately be framed by "the doctrine of human rights that asserts that human dignity is intrinsic to, and the basis of all human rights."

The role of faith and religion

However, when it came to threading the needle of what comprised morality and what constituted faith, the eye of the needle suddenly seemed very narrow. As Cochrane explained:

The HIV movement in South Africa is one largely belatedly taken on by the faith community. People of faith no longer had to battle the apartheid state, but now they had to recognize this new threat to our society. It was hard. Precisely when we thought we were going to build a new society, we were facing a new threat, now from a disease. As the post-Apartheid state began to stumble around HIV and AIDS, activists begin to find their energy to get behind this new struggle.

But many had been linked to the United Democratic Front,[2] and not many were the religious folks. In fact, the religious community, the faith community, including those strongly involved against apartheid, found it quite difficult to deal with this new phenomenon, partly because religious movements had become weaker in the post-apartheid situation. Then they knew what they were against, yet not really quite what they were *for*, so there was a loss of identity, and, a quite serious loss of focus, except perhaps among those most directly infected or affected by HIV.

Initially, for people of faith it was a real battle, partly because of the issue of sexuality, which has always been problematic for faith communities, and particularly because it was also attached to same-sex relations very early on – a major difficulty for many in the faith community. There was in a sense a paralysis, in the Christian community at least, though the Muslim community has had difficulties too.

However, this changed gradually over time, as Cochrane noted, "Statements from the gay and lesbian community, and people such as the well-known HIV and gay-rights activist and Justice of the Constitutional Court of South Africa, Edwin Cameron, made a huge difference. Early, initial statements about HIV by Nelson Mandela also made a difference, though matters became confused under Thabo Mbeki and his health minister, Manto Tshabalala-Msimang."

The struggle around HIV and AIDS was a striving for social justice and inclusivity in a country where these constructs had been in short supply over the ages, and long denied to so many. From a theological standpoint, it was the inner quest to be a decent human being, and to act accordingly to others, irrespective of differences beyond the fact of being human—a categorical imperative in which there are no grey areas, no 'lesser' human beings.

Farid Esack is a South African Islamic scholar and, through Positive Muslims, an HIV activist. Cochrane's narrative is reminiscent of these thoughts on the role of religion in society: "Beyond the façade of difference there is a common humanity. If religion loses sight of that it becomes a negative, if not a demonic, force in society." Esack argues that the need to see beyond our particular faith, tradition, culture and status in life is perhaps the toughest assignment that life can throw at us. It requires us to divest ourselves of the presuppositions of race, gender, religion and class that sometimes make us less than human, allowing us to think we are superior to those who are different from us.[3]

Esack's view echoes Cochrane's point that while "by and large the religious community" had at first failed, this was not true of those "many religious people of faith on the ground, especially the women who had to look after the sick people." They faced death daily, and they did not fall short. "So the transition from human rights activism to that of HIV takes place among certain groups of people who feel directly affected by the disease. It is no coincidence that people like Zackie Achmat [who co-founded the Treatment Action Campaign] is now involved in other issues related to human rights, beyond HIV. It is a natural extension."

Cochrane, like Esack, sees religion as having the capacity to make us better human beings. "The condition of possibility of being human – the necessary assumption we must make in order to understand what characterizes us in a way and to a degree that is true of no other animal as far as we know – is our capacity for creative freedom. That capacity is intrinsically good, not in the sense of morality, but as the condition of our being." He quotes activist Steve Biko: "Freedom is the ability to define oneself with one's possibilities held back not by the power of other people over one but only by one's relationship to God and to natural surroundings."

A moral imperative

The human rights debate remains one that is complicated and complex. It raises questions that cannot be answered by the usual constellation of responses. Not a few people argue, critically, that human rights discourse is merely an extension of Western ideals. Cochrane thinks that "we need to be more nuanced than that," recognizing at the heart of this discourse that the affirmation of human dignity is not culturally specific. Moreover, popular dichotomies between "West and the rest" (or "South" versus "North") are not accurate descriptions of what he refers to as "the interwoven nests of asymmetrical power and knowledge that not only straddle national and cultural boundaries, but also occur within them."

How do we address such asymmetries and their injustices? Cochrane turns again to:

> the extraordinary capacity we as human beings have to add to nature or what does not already exist, to not only grasp the way nature works, but to transform it in ways that no other creature that we know of, is capable of doing. This extraordinarily powerful capacity enables us to make inventions with which we can destroy other, even blow the entire world up; but, crucially, it also enables us to build societies that match the highest of which we are capable. This is our calling.

Cochrane's view of religion is related:

> It rests upon an understanding of "religion" (as a universal aspect of human being) that is closely tied in to the notion of human rights in relation to human dignity and human capacities. Usually, when we say "religion," we mean specific, historical, cultural expressions or traditions. That is not what I mean here. For such specific expressions/traditions I now reserve the word "faith" or "faiths," This enables me to explain why I see "religion" a universal human dimension of being, and also why faiths, which are clearly particular and, as such, often caught up in defending their particularity, can be both good and bad.

For Cochrane, this is what compels us to fight against what might "rightly be called evil," which he argues, like Biko and Frantz Fanon, we can define as that which "diminishes or destroys humanity."

> It is not a coincidence that for most of us our heroes or models of what it means to live a life worth living are precisely those who exhibit a capability, even in the most dire circumstances, to transcend their self-interest in the interest of all and of the whole. They represent the highest of which we, too, are capable. Properly understood, this is the core of religion . . . The point is not to deny the importance of particular traditions, but to recognize both their limits and the vital elements within them that help us towards that core: the call to live up to the highest of which we are capable, to give our lives, if you like, to life.

Questions for discussion

• How would you define "being human" from a faith perspective, and how can you link this to dignity and social justice?

Chapter 11

"Let Grace Be Total": The Ministry of the United Church of Christ in the Philippines

Erlinda N. Senturias

The United Church of Christ in the Philippines (UCCP) of which I am a member is an affirming, welcoming, accepting and, caring faith community. Our reformed theology is based on grace that manifests in our desired goal of promoting human dignity, human rights, justice, peace, integrity, and freedom. For example, the stance of our church on the issue of lesbian, gay, bisexual, and transsexual is "**Let Grace Be Total.**" Our faith tradition affirms that "we consider the grace of God as an unconditional gift of God." We believe in God's healing and reconciling love and that God sent our Lord Jesus Christ to be "in humble solidarity with the lost, the last and the least in this world." It is consistent with our understanding of the radical and evangelical perspectives of the New Testament gospels and letters to the early Christian churches.

It is clear in the statement that "we worship and follow a God who in the spirit of this great love for all took the most unthinkable and so radical step for a powerful, divine being to undertake, to humble Himself and stand in complete solidarity with the most ordinary, powerless, alienated and struggling people of this world."[1]

In the same spirit, the UCCP Cosmopolitan Church has been engaged in the HIV ministry since 2013 with both human rights and human dignity perspectives rooted in the theology of grace and freedom as the underlying theological principles. As a local church, we have so much to overcome from our own culture of shame, stigma, and judgmentalism derived from some fundamentalist teachings that were imbibed in the past and continue to be a source of debate. Despite the controversies within the church, the HIV ministry addresses stigma, shame, denial, discrimination, inaction, and mis-action (SSDDIM) as a way to educate members of our congregation on HIV prevention and human rights promotion. It is also a way to make our church open to engaging with people living with HIV and AIDS. We can provide meaningful involvement and safe spaces for our very own people living with HIV to exercise leadership in the ministry, as well as for those personally affected to champion HIV where human dignity, grace, and freedom are embraced and given full expression.

Chapter 12

Stigma, HIV, and Diverse Sexuality: Examples of Faith Responses Affirming Human Dignity

JP Mokgethi-Heath

"The global response to HIV has once again reminded us to be the church it is called to be; a responsive church that stands with the voiceless and down trodden – a church which has identified itself with the most affected population, giving them the voice and being in the forefront of contributing to the search or solutions to end the epidemic and its subsequent vulnerabilities than being passive recipients of charity. Moving forward, the church is being challenged if not compelled to soul search, looking at how we can further maximize our efforts (even if it means challenging our own comfort), and redefine our theological approaches that perpetuate exclusion as approaches

that are inclusive, characterized by solidarity so as to leave
no one behind."
　　—Rev. Canon MacDonald S. Sembereka, Executive
　　　　Director, Global Interfaith Network on Sex, Sexual
　　　　Orientation, Gender Identity and Expression

Challenges related to stigma, discrimination, and service delivery for people living with HIV are an everyday occurrence. People encounter them when they visit the dentist, who says, "I can't help you during the day, I will lose all my patients"; or when they seek work in the police service or military, where they are told, "As a person with AIDS you simply are not strong enough to work in this job"; or when they try to acquire medicine and hear, "We have a challenge in terms of medication: we can only give you five days medication. Come back again then." These daily challenges are even more acute for people with diverse sexuality.

During the 2012 International Congress on AIDS in Asia and Pacific (ICAAP), research was presented on the Syndemic Construct[1] for Men who have Sex with Men (MSM). The study looked at six different situations for MSMs, and found that in more than one of them, the syndemic impact increased a negative self-image. Such an impact reduced the likelihood of people considering themselves worthy of HIV prevention or –for those who test positive – worthy of seeking treatment. The six situations mentioned were: being rejected by family on the grounds of sexual orientation; having attempted suicide; being rejected by faith community on the grounds of sexual orientation; having abused substances; having done sex work; and being physically, physiologically, or sexually abused in a relationship

What is clear is that all of the six situations described above are areas in which the faith community can have a positive impact. Here we can be the voice that affirms people instead of the voice that breaks people down. The reality check, however, is that this affirmation is too frequently not experienced by those who need it the most. The increased vulnerability related both to HIV transmission and to HIV-related morbidity and mortality forces us to reflect on the engagement of faith communities in this regard.

Strong resistance from a number of countries to issues of human sexuality, and more particularly homosexuality, has usually been justified by religious beliefs. Clear examples of this come from Uganda and Kenya, where faith community leaders have spoken out in favour of "law reform" that would signal a step backward for human rights, and would further burden homosexual people in terms of both vulnerability to HIV and access to HIV-related prevention, treatment, care, and support. In these settings, faith communities have spoken about viewing members of the LGBTI community as people who have rejected biblical values and are anti-cultural. Clearly work is needed to help shift the paradigm of current understanding on human sexuality.

I will highlight three examples of positive involvement with faith that offer opportunities for different engagement in this regard:

The International Lesbian and Gay Association (ILGA)

The ILGA was first formed as the International Gay Association in 1978. While LGBTI groups have long worked to engage the UN and countries internationally on issues related to the human rights of LGBTI people, there was no faith input in this campaign. During the 2012 ILGA conference in Stockholm, members of the LGBTI community who also identified themselves as people of faith expressed the need to form a network of LGBTI people and allies within faith communities who could identify and develop material to help these communities engage with issues on human sexuality. As a result, in January 2014, the Global Interfaith Network for People of all Sexes, Sexual Orientations, Gender Identities and Expressions (GIN-SSOGIE) was formed. In October 2014, in Mexico City, GIN-SSOGIE, for the first time, led a pre-conference to the ILGA Conference, one that 100 of the 500 conference delegates attended.

Bangalore Interfaith Declaration on Homophobia

Inclusive and affirming notions related to sexual orientation are at times seen as secular, European, and even anti-faith and anti-family. Working with issues of human sexuality in African or Asian contexts becomes very difficult when messages of inclusion are seen as a challenge to everything held dear. The value of this type of work done outside of Europe or America is inestimable, as this can be seen as a more authentic faith response. A wonderful example is the Bangalore Interfaith Declaration on Homophobia made in May 2014. I want to quote a single paragraph to give an idea of the engaging language used:

> We observe that religions play significant roles in the Indian society in the
> ethical discernment of their adherents. Scriptures, traditions, moral codes,

and practices form and formulate religious teachings and ethics on personal and social life. However, religious traditions tend to interpret these rich sources and resources to legitimize dominant notions of truth and morality. Such attempts unfortunately legitimize moral codes that are unjust and condemn and demonize people who transgress the dominant norms because of their convictions. Homophobia is one such reality, where sexual minorities are constructed as immoral based on hetero-normativity. As a result, homosexuals and transgenders are often rejected and shunned by religious and faith based organizations. This situation calls for deeper introspection and transformation so that religions will abstain from sowing the seeds of bigotry and homophobia, and instead promote dignity, inclusivity, and equality, while accepting, respecting and celebrating differences.[2]

Uppsala Festival of Theology

An Uppsala Festival of Theology is convened in Sweden every three years. It brings together more than 1000 theologians engaging in various streams. In February 2015, an LGBTI stream was preceded by three days of dialogue. The dialogue included five people from each of the three Abrahamic faiths. Through a partnership with GIN-SSOGIE, three theologians – one each from the Jewish, Christian, and Muslim faiths – were identified. They developed resource packs showing methodologies of reading sacred texts in ways that were more authentic or engaging. They demonstrated that at the very least no one of the Abrahamic faiths could justify the persecution of people on the grounds of their sexual orientation. Face-to-face dialogue between people of faith, both from the LGBTI community and from outside of it, led to a deep respect for each other. They were able to issue a statement calling for expanded dialogue:

> We felt greatly deepened and enriched by this interfaith dialogue. It created for us a renewed sense of responsibility and accountability, and instilled a sense of urgency to create safe spaces in our communities and in our world. Hence, we call for the dialogue to be continued and expanded within and between our faith communities and the wider society.[3]

Affirming human dignity, showing the links between human dignity and human rights, and attempting to identify the prejudices that we ourselves bring to our reading of scripture are crucial steps in finding ways to build self-esteem and to remove some of the factors that increase people's vulnerability to HIV.

Questions for discussion

- Is your faith community a place where people of diverse sexualities can feel welcome? Why might this be important?

Chapter 13

A Common Language for Human Rights, Faith, and HIV: An Example of Ministry in the Philippines

Richard R. Mickley

Ecumenical ministry in relation to HIV and AIDS

How can we find a common language for human rights, faith, and HIV? For over 40 years, I have worked with people living with HIV. Preaching, teaching and writing, I have worked in three environments: in Los Angeles, where we did everything we could for friends who were dying of a mysterious disease whose name we did not yet know; in interfaith ministry in New Zealand; and now, today, in the Philippines, where we have developed the Well Wellness Method, which provides direct, holistic help to people living with HIV. In each of these contexts, I have found myself struggling with the question: What is the role of ecumenical ministry in creating an informed, safe, and enabling environment to reduce stigma and improve access to health and other services?

This is not the approach of those many people of faith who, faced by HIV, will sit in judgment over human beings who do not follow their own rules. NO masturbation, they say; NO condoms; NO sex except to make babies.

And NO sex through your whole life if you are attracted to the same sex. Every one of these "mandates" can produce trauma. In fact, many of my 40-plus years in ecumenical ministry have been spent holding the hands of wounded people who are in bondage to these prohibitions. And many of the most wounded are those living with HIV. Men and women both suffer, but the stigma is compounded when it is directed at men who have sex with men and at transgender people.

So what is an authentic ministry in this situation, and how should we speak about human rights in a manner that affirms religious authenticity? At the Well, we are motivated by at least three beautiful passages from the gospels. The first is the story in John 4 about Jesus meeting a woman at a well: a meeting where he gave the life-changing promise, "The water I will give shall be a well of water springing up into everlasting life." The second is Jesus' story in Luke 10 of the wounded man, bleeding by the roadside, who is ignored by a priest on his way to the temple to pray. The hero of this story is a rejected "heretic," a man hated by the religion of Jesus, Joseph, and Mary. But Jesus held him up as the hero, not because of his religion, but because of his caring and human concern for a man who may have been dying. We now call this person the Good Samaritan. The third is the profound scriptural statement: "What you did for the least of these, you did for me" (Matt. 25).

So, what is an authentic role for the church in the context of this ecumenical ministry?

The ecumenical ministry of the Well is authentic in that we and our wonderful staff make the Well Method available in bringing together people, faith, and science to conquer HIV and achieve the fulfilled life God's people were created to enjoy. And that, surely, is social justice in action: creating an informed, safe, and enabling environment to reduce stigma and improve access to health and other services.

Wellness: A truly Christian ministry

When church teaching is used to promote stigma, then it represents an unjust and ugly turning away from the way of Jesus. Ecumenical ministry must reverse this ugly way. The church, the churches, and orders like Maryknoll have been committed Good Samaritans. So what is lacking? Those who work in the ministry of the Well are people who have faith in the way of caring and healing that Jesus lived out and recommended. They do not believe this because it is the faith of the wounded: that is irrelevant. They follow Jesus *because that is our faith.*

At the Well, we have no charge, no fee, no salary. Our focus is entirely on the person who is now living with HIV. They need wellness. No matter how much money, time, effort, and money are spent on social and societal infrastructure, those three scriptures speak of a person-to-person relationship within a caring, healing, affirming ministry to people living with HIV. When global strategy is discussed, we should never forget this bottom line. We need prevention and testing, but we also need wellness. The Well Method deals with all the wounds that people living with HIV have experienced.

So the Well Method is not a place. The Well Method is not for sale. It can be learned and applied anywhere in the world to guide people living with HIV to a life of wellness and fulfilment – mutually and joyfully supporting each other in doing so. Whether it's North or South, in this arena we don't see the phenomena of North-South tension; we see the same phenomenon of stigmatized people who have been driven underground, who have been deprived by people of faith from adhering to the faith that once was theirs, and who come back again to life.

Many of them have suffered at the hands of religious people. For example, so-called followers may ascribe to their god messages like, "I will love you if . . . you don't love the one you love." Such a god is surely not really God, especially if the followers urge hatred and even kill in that god's name. With a common language of unity and justice, people everywhere can build a better world, wherever they are, by embracing the way of a God of unconditional love. The real God is a god of peace and love.

Just recently it was reported that a 16-year-old boy in Colombia was outed by the principal of his Christian high school after they saw a photo on his cell phone of him kissing his boyfriend. They ridiculed and harassed him till they found his suicide note:

> *Goodbye cruel world*
> *I'm leaving you today*
> *Goodbye*
> *Goodbye*
> *Goodbye*
> *Goodbye all you people*
> *There's nothing you can say*

To make me change
My mind
Goodbye.

For that's what stigma does. Some leave family; some leave church; some just leave this world. Everywhere people living with HIV suffer from stigma, which undermines healthcare programs and causes untold suffering. In our country, an October 2014 report from the Philippine Department of Health noted that as many as two-thirds of people living with HIV are prevented by fear of stigma from seeking medical help. The report urged people living with HIV to care for their health and work for their own survival. Yet how many, because of stigma, are so afraid of HIV testing that they resist the knowledge that they are HIV positive?

Toward a solution?

How will the world save its stigmatized, traumatized "sexual minorities"? It will surely require concerted worldwide efforts. And then, within that wider agenda, what can the faith community do to reverse practices of injustice and enhance social justice? The answer, in Jesus' words and in Christian teaching, is love. So for years, despite all that has been seen and said about the churches' non-observance of human rights, some faith communities have been doing wonderful, authentic, ecumenical ministry.

In my ministry alone, I have experienced numerous examples. For a start, I have experienced the affirming ecumenical ministry of the Metropolitan Community Churches worldwide. Then, I served as coordinator of a wonderful ecumenical initiative of the National Council of Churches in New Zealand, designed to develop a "manifesto for caring Christian ministry to persons with HIV," avoiding sex-negative theology, and practising empathic ministry with sex-positive theology. Those clergy who signed the statement received referrals for providing affirming Christian ministry. The Catholic Dioceses of One Spirit, wherever its priests are present around the world, provide an ecumenical refuge for divorced persons and all those seeking true Christ-like Christian ministry free of prejudice, homophobia, and condemnation.

Now, of course, we see this on a much larger scale among many of the organizations, for instance, in the Ecumenical Advocacy Alliance and their common vision of justice, dignity, and life. Can that ministry be further expanded, I wonder? Is it possible that Jesus' prayer "that they be one" – offered for his own followers – might one day become a reality? For the way of Jesus is not denial of hope, destruction of faith, nor demolition of self-esteem. What could be further from human rights? The way of Jesus is to be truly ecumenical, to be one, in the one Spirit. Like the woman at the well, a person living with HIV experiences a changed life when the way of unity and justice becomes the path to wellbeing and fulfilment.

Question for discussion

- What do you consider to be the church's role in creating an informed, safe, and enabling environment, particularly when addressing issues of sex and sexuality?

Chapter 14

As Science Advances . . . the Human Heart Hardens: A Brazilian Perspective

Ester Lisboa

"Create in me, O God, a pure heart and renew in me a
steadfast spirit."
– Ps. 51:10

Questioning our certainties

The United Nations' goal is to end the HIV epidemic by 2030.[1] This does not mean the extinction of the virus, but the reduction of numbers of those infected. The interim treatment target is that by 2020, 90 percent of all people living with HIV will know their HIV status; 90 percent of all people with diagnosed HIV infection will receive sustained antiretroviral therapy; 90 percent of all people receiving antiretroviral therapy will have viral suppression. This treatment target – referred to as "90-90-90" – appears difficult to achieve. However, the response to the epidemic has generated a global movement of solidarity, protest, and demonstration that has transformed how we address issues of health and development, and as a result many in the scientific community think that these targets are possible. Nearly 35 years into the epidemic, AIDS is no longer mysterious, and efforts to fight it are achieving results

But is the whole answer to be found in science? AIDS continues victimizing men, women, and young people who are exposed to religiously justified discrimination and stigmatization. It sometimes seems it will be easier to produce a vaccine against AIDS than to regenerate the hearts of many people who identify themselves as people of faith.

So why are HIV and AIDS not always dealt with impartially, accurately, or comprehensively among people of faith? The respectability that faith communities inspire and the social capital they hold have the capacity to play a strategic role in preventing HIV and in disseminating information. Where prejudice and discrimination are justified by a pseudo-religious morality, our faith communities should be able to join in the fight against them.

Fabio Mesquita is director of the Sexual Transmitted Diseases (STD) / AIDS Department of the Ministry of Health of Brazil. This national institution, he says, is in line with the United Nations target. "If we continue with all essential work to combat the epidemic, we can reduce the levels," he claims. For Ricardo Diaz, expert on infectious disease of the Federal University of São Paulo, the public health message is simple:

> The more people who do the test and detect the virus, the more will seek treatment early on. Transmission is always proportional to the amount of virus that the person has in the blood. If the use of drugs has the expected success, the viral load becomes undetectable, the infection decreases and we will not have new cases of AIDS.[2]

Therefore, religious communities are faced with the challenge of working, seriously and responsibly, to address the stigma and taboo that are still associated with HIV and AIDS. We cannot continue falling into errors of omission. We need to deal with the existence of misinformation, and the lack of understanding in faith groups that sexuality is God's gift. This will not be easy: it is a fact that the reality of AIDS makes us question our certainties, and that is always uncomfortable.

Faith communities in Brazil

Brazil is a country of many religious traditions, notably Christianity, Islam, African-Brazilian, and Judaism. This diversity is the result of a series of migratory movements, which included the forced migration or trafficking of enslaved people from the African continent. Dialogue between these highly diverse inter-religious and ecumenical population can be of great help to faith-based organizations in overcoming prejudice and taboos.

Brazil has always been at the forefront of the AIDS movement, promoting an innovative approach based on strong political commitment, scientific evidence, and human rights principles. National response is inclusive, with the strategic role of governments at various levels and of sectors such as academia, civil society organizations (including people living with HIV), the private sector, international partners, and religious communities.

Brazil's National Council of Christian Churches (CONIC) is one of the organizations represented in CNAIDS, the country's coordinating committee on STD, AIDS and Viral Hepatitis. CONIC's mission is "to be at the service of the unity of the churches, striving to accompany the Brazilian reality, confronting it with the Gospel and the demands of the Reign of God." It is the commitment of CONIC, therefore, to act in favour of people's dignity, rights, and duties. One of its objectives is to promote ecumenical relations between the Christian churches and to strengthen the common witness of member churches in the defence of human rights. Hence, its presence in CNAIDS supports a specific and prophetic perspective regarding prevention, care, and access to treatment.

For that to be a reality, an important goal is to reduce stigma and discrimination. The epidemic exposes religion's silence and indifference to some forms of suffering, and the prejudice and discrimination this produces. At the same time, it challenges churches to become better informed and engaged in the work of reconciliation.

There are strong parallels between this reality and the biblical story about God's experience of regret, in Genesis:

> The Lord saw how great the wickedness of the human race had become on the earth, and that every inclination of the thoughts of the human heart was only evil all the time. The Lord regretted that he had made human beings on the earth, and his heart was deeply troubled. So the Lord said, "I will wipe from the face of the earth the human race I have created—and with them the

animals, the birds and the creatures that move along the ground—for I regret that I have made them. (Gen. 6: 5-7)

Surely God is troubled by the sight of young people who are being infected while their schools refuse to allow HIV prevention to be mentioned within their walls, forbid teaching about condoms, and ban participation in the HPV (Human Papilloma Virus) prevention campaign.

Toward a commitment

Surely God is also troubled by the experience of persons who, having lived with AIDS for 25 years, continue to suffer prejudice, stigma, and rejection, amounting to "civil death," at the hands of a conservative, ruthless, and judgmental society. AIDS in Brazil is not just a medical epidemic: it is also a social one.

Did God regret having created human kind in general? NO! God was saddened by the realization that human evil had reached such proportions. God has no pleasure in the death of anyone. The Genesis story is a direct expression of God's grief. Here in Brazil, I believe God grieves because the intrinsic dignity of every human being has been disregarded. The struggle for recognition of the dignity of all people is a duty to be lived out every day.

To put this into practice is to exercise solidarity with those who suffer from the disease and to act against all forms of discrimination. Sometimes it seems that we live in a society where joy has given way to fear, love to hatred, solidarity to indifference, and union to separation. In relation to HIV and AIDS, we too often find ourselves, today, living in a society that criminalizes affection, love, happiness.

So, as people of faith, we are called to fulfil our obligation of honouring the human dignity of all people. In watching us living out greater love in our graced communities, God could cease to grieve. God, instead, could be proud of God's creatures.

Questions for discussion

- This essay mentions some international targets for ending the HIV epidemic. In relation to your own context, are these realistic? If not, how can faith communities help meet them?

Chapter 15

The Armenian Apostolic Church: An Orthodox Church's Response to the Challenges of HIV and AIDS

Karine Kocharian

A difficult call

Around 95 percent of Armenians are Christians, and most of these belong to the Armenian Apostolic Church. So in 1988, when Armenia's first cases of HIV were registered, the church was one of the first institutions people turned to. At the time, a diagnosis of HIV or AIDS was thought of as a death sentence. People came to the church asking, "Is this a manifestation of God's wrath against sinners?" Or they asked, "If God is responsible for this calamity, does it mean our loving God is in fact an angry, punishing God?" "In a time of AIDS," they asked, "where do we find hope?" So Christian churches found themselves facing demands for theological answers, as well as for practical support. It was a difficult call, posing theological and ethical dilemmas that related to health and health care, social organization and family life.

Since then, clergy and others have responded to the challenge of those early days. They have provided practical support to people living with HIV and AIDS and their families, made their teaching more accessible to lay people, and learned to avoid language and scriptural interpretations that can lead to the stigmatization of people living with or affected by HIV. One example of this is the association, often made, between HIV transmission and sin. This was a difficult issue for the leadership to address. The mission of the church, they thought, was to heal people through nurturing an environment in which Orthodox understandings of morality and freedom were maintained. But violations of Divine Law do involve a concept of sin, and they had no wish to question important areas of moral teaching.

In particular, the challenge of HIV gave rise to a new direction of diaconal work, with the Armenian Church leadership emphasizing the distinctive role that the church has to play on individual and societal levels. The leadership, therefore, ran seminars and training courses. They also brought speakers from other churches, including the Russian Orthodox Church and Protestant churches, to prepare Armenian church clergy to provide proper quality service to people living with HIV and their communities. It is the church's primary responsibility, they said, to provide spiritual and moral support and care to people with HIV in their darkest times, when the normal pace of life is disrupted by thoughts of disability and death, anxiety about the future, and isolation from society.

The church is called, also, to be a steward of society's moral and cultural values and norms. Where prejudice and ignorance contribute to HIV-related stigma or discrimination, the church must seek to foster a more caring and accepting atmosphere, and to encourage a spirituality and a sense of moral responsibility that will contribute to HIV prevention. A step-by-step approach was implemented to prepare priests for this mission in their communities.

Human values are Christian values

In 2009, under the leadership of Fr Grigor Grigoryan, the Armenian Round Table Interchurch Foundation established a Day Centre for people living with HIV. This centre was a joint venture between the Armenian Apostolic Church and "Real Life, Real World," an NGO of people living with HIV. Fr Grigor recalls his early days as director of the entre. People then were not open to discussion. The lack of trust was apparent. Yet the longing to be truly heard and acknowledged was stronger. After a short while, after several group meetings with the priest, the number of beneficiaries who asked for individual counselling grew.

Since 2011 the Day Centre has been operating under the auspices of the Araratyan Pontifical Diocese as one of the church's biggest specialized charity centres. At present, it serves about 700 people who are in need of moral-psychological support, including about 350 people living with HIV, 150 HIV-affected children and youth, 17 people who inject drugs, and more than 100 family members who are in need of moral-psychological support. These come not only from the area of Araratyan Diocese but from any region of Armenia.

Social marginalization, isolation from society, personality crisis, and multiple anxieties are the foci of the work that the Day Centre carries out on daily basis; and through years of experience, the centre has developed and implemented a comprehensive approach and a full set of services. Trained personnel, including professionals and peer-to-peer staff, work hand-in-hand with the Christian priest to provide moral and psychological support. Clients are helped through individual or group encounters, or by phone consultations with the psychologist, social worker, peer-to peer consultants, and other staff and volunteers. Day care for children and vocational training courses for Day Centre clients help improve the social-economic situation of the families, and direct humanitarian aid is provided monthly to those most in need.

At the core of the service is the non-judgmental spiritual and moral support the priests provide to people living with HIV and their families. However, there is no compulsion for visitors to engage with its Christian motivation. The centre is there to serve any person who needs psychological and social support, regardless of where they are in their spiritual journey in the given moment. People of any faith or none are welcome to use its services.

"Paradise Family"

The Armenian Apostolic Church has always believed that the institution of the family plays a uniquely important role in a person's spiritual, moral and social development. The concept of a "Paradise Family" was coined by one of the patriarchs of Armenian Church, the brilliant theologian, Catholicos of all Armenians. Mkrtich Khrimyan is affectionately known as Mkrtich Hayrig (Mkrtich, the father of the nation). His image of the Paradise Family became the cornerstone for work with people living with HIV, many of whom come to the Day Centre not just in poor physical and psychological condition, but also alienated from their families. Along with the leader-priest, Day Centre staff try to reach out to those families and to educate them on how to overcome the misinformation and fear they associate with their relative's HIV-positive status, and to encourage them to provide the care and support that is so desperately needed. In this ministry to families, social workers and priests pay home visits, invite relatives to friendly conversations, and welcome them to visit the Day Centre and talk about their concerns. Today, there are family members who have become full-fledged clients of the Day Centre, using the services of the psychologist or of the social worker, who directs them tactfully to health or other services that can be of help to the HIV-positive relative.

The success of the Day Centre must to a certain extent be attributed to the fact that so many of its activities and services are led and developed by people who are themselves living with HIV. We see peer-to-peer consultants working hand-in-hand with the professional staff and clergy, mutually educating each other on the sensitive issues of the work. Many volunteers of the centre have felt empowered to take on the role of mentor to people who have recently had a positive diagnosis.

Another major success story of the Day Centre is its work with people living with HIV who were injecting drug users. With the priest's spiritual guidance and moral support, most of them have successfully started a life free from drugs and are working toward a fulfilling lifestyle, taking each day as it comes. This group of recovering people who inject drugs has become a faithful following within the church, attending not only for services but in order to volunteer for various charity and construction projects. This type of work greatly aids their recovery, allowing them to re-gain the sense of belonging to a community and also a feeling that they are capable of doing something for others: an experience of new life that many have described as re-inventing themselves.

Work with children and youth

About 15 children living with HIV and 150 HIV-affected children and adolescents attend the Day Centre either occasionally or on regular basis. Some of these children are paternal orphans whose fathers have died of AIDS, leaving the families in extreme poverty. Most of the children who come to the centre have either both or one parent with an HIV-positive status. The services they are offered are well-rounded, including direct social assistance to families, the professional services of a psychologist, and diverse cultural and educational programs aimed at contributing to their confidence-building and meeting their needs for education.

The Day Centre – with its trusting, accepting, and caring atmosphere – is therefore considered by its beneficiaries as "a safe home" for people living with HIV, people who inject drugs, and their families. Here they can share their thoughts, concerns, and joy. This "safe home" is not another place for isolation, but a secure ground where people can find an inner peace, a point of balance, and the confidence to go on with their lives outside of the walls of the Day Centre.

Prevention, fighting stigma, and discrimination

At present, in Armenia, there is no lack of HIV information campaigns. However, interestingly enough, ignorance and lack of applied knowledge are still huge problems. The church considers it a priority to guide its faith communities toward a better understanding of the personal responsibility they must take for their own lives, and their responsibility to other people. Preventive actions include sermons and seminars led by priests working in the communities. These usually include a priest talking to his community on the topics of family relationships, moral principles that are central to Christian living, and the importance of respect toward one's own body as God's temple. This will be accompanied by input on the basic facts about HIV and AIDS, sometimes provided by a health specialist or a volunteer living with HIV.

Held both with adults and with teenagers, these meetings sometimes include innovative challenges to self-expression that may include writing essays and making posters and artwork. The hope is that this creative experience may have a bigger emotional impact and bring forth attitude and behavioural changes. One example is *LadYa,* is an educational methodology developed at the Russian Orthodox Church. Adapted for an Armenian cultural context, the training course is used to encourage youth to develop an overall Christian-like attitude to life, where decisions ideally derive from feelings of love, compassion, and a sense of responsibility and ownership over the life choices they make.

Conclusion

Fr Grigor Grigoryan, the director of the Day Centre, tells a story about a client who was also an injecting drug user. During an individual session, this person said to him, "I am happy I have HIV." "Why?" asked the priest, amazed. "Because HIV brought me to God and to a more purposeful life," answered his client.

There is no doubt that the church and its communities have gone through many changes in the light of the HIV epidemic. The church itself has developed the quality of its services, and the communities have succeeded in overcoming much of the stigma attached to HIV and AIDS. The latter have been helped by a clear explanation of the deed-consequence approach to HIV, as opposed to a sin-punishment view. The growing number of people living with HIV and AIDS-related complications has also forced change. This is not an abstract problem, but one that is deeply tangible in our society. At the same time there remain challenges and struggles. Paramount among these is the difficulty of engaging more effectively with men, particularly those who find themselves caught up in poor economic conditions and are forced to find seasonal work abroad.

The Armenian Apostolic Church has an exceptional role to play in easing the pain of people living with HIV and helping them to heal their lives and the lives of their families. As a result, the church is highly appreciated not only by people living with HIV, but also by the relevant healthcare institutions. Due to its careful movement forward, the church has developed a solid body of experience and conceptualized knowledge, which is documented in the draft concept of the church on issues of HIV/AIDS. This concept paper serves as a guide for servants of the church when confronted by the various ethical dilemmas they meet in their everyday service in the communities. And so the church has developed a way of working that honours the basic dignity of all human beings as full and equal members of God's family.

Questions for discussion

- The phrase "human rights" has not been used in this essay. Nevertheless, the day centre's work is underpinned by a profound understanding of human dignity. Have you ever encountered resistance to the language of human rights? Might there be a case for developing different ways of talking about these issues?

Chapter 16

Living by Faith in Challenging Times: A Caribbean View on What It Means to Say, "God Will Take Care of Us"

Garth Minott

What does it mean to say that God will take care of us?

A few years ago, I was at a church office and had just completed a counselling session with a young man who was living with HIV.[1] A member of the church arrived to see me just as I emerged from the office with Andrew (not his real name). When I extended my hand to shake the member's hand, she pulled away. She had come to see me, she said, but upon finding me in the company of Andrew she never wished to see me again. Furthermore, she would never return to the church office, as she might have to sit in the chair Andrew had previously sat on, and she did not want to be contaminated. This church-member was a Christian. Like the person of faith, in chapters 1 and 2 of the Book of Wisdom, I felt ridiculed. But I also somehow felt that God would take care of her, of Andrew and me.

So what is going on here?

We are living, today, in challenging times: just like the people to whom the Book of Wisdom was addressed. Written around the second century before Jesus was born, this wonderful book reflects a people at a point of transition in their journey of faith. Their ancestors had been slaves in Egypt. They had been forced into exile in Babylon. Still the political climate was uncertain, with the Roman general Pompey moving steadily through the Mediterranean area and claiming territory after territory. So for the Jewish people, this was a time of uncertainty about how the future would unfold. Yet here, in this reading, we find the writer saying to the people, "God will take care of you."

Now the incident I described above took place in early 2000, just before the Jamaican government took the decision to cover the full cost of medication for those living with HIV. With such medication available, people could live for a long time with HIV. Today, though, the government has found that it cannot cover the full cost of HIV medication for all those who need it, and consequently only about 80 percent of those who need it will receive it. The other 20 percent are given whatever is needed to keep them comfortable until they die. So that, whether they are on HIV medication regimens or not, the message to all those who are infected or affected by HIV and AIDS is that "God will take care of you."

But back to my story. Although Andrew was not a Christian, I had met him through two members of the church who decided, on their own, to sponsor his medication. However, it was very important that Andrew maintained a healthy emotional, physical and spiritual life. "God will take care of you," was the message I was sharing with him during our weekly meetings.

This was no light thing to say, any more than it was for the writer of the Book of Wisdom, to reassure God's people that God would take care of them. That was 200 years before Jesus was born. And yet the message of the resurrection was at the heart of what its writer wanted to convey. We see that already the idea of resurrection was taking root in the minds and hearts of the people of God. It was this doctrine of the resurrection that Jesus took as his own, built on, taught his followers about, and finally manifested it in his own life, death, and resurrection from the dead. At the heart of this message of resurrection was the assurance that God would take care of God's people.

The meaning of the resurrection, then, is that nothing in this life has the final say. As St Paul puts it, "Neither death nor life nor angels not principalities nor things in heaven nor things on earth can separate us from the love of God in Christ Jesus our Lord" (Rom. 8:38-39). Of course as people of God we will have to encounter various challenges in our lives. We are assured, though, that it is not those challenges that define who we are. Rather, it is the fact that God takes care of us that is the message of the resurrection. That is the road map for guiding the people of faith, the guiding principle I took with me as I met with Andrew week after week to assure him that he is not alone in his journey.

He did feel lonely and abandoned. But week by week I assured him that the God who created him would not abandon him. And week by week he described encounters with people in the community who beat him, spat on him, and insulted him. Apart from his mother, who sadly died before him, even his family members wanted nothing to do with him. Listening to his story it pained my heart to hear what Martin Luther King Jr described as "man's inhumanity to man."

A public health issue

Andrew's story made it clear to me that we urgently need prophets of compassion to be able to assert that God cares for people. And this message of caring cannot just be words: it has to be accompanied by action. Recently, in conducting a focus group discussion, I was present when the following conversation took place.

An Anglican, who was working for the Jamaican government as a public health nurse, described three challenges she faced as a person of faith working with the Ministry of Health. First, as a person of faith she wondered what her Anglican Church would think of her if they saw her meeting with sex workers and men who have sex with men (MSM), talking with them about safe sex and the need to use a condom. She wondered how realistic some of her fellow church members were as they made pronouncements concerning these "dirty, good for nothing people."

Second, she is aware of the government's concern to maintain effective public health measures. Yet, on the other hand, public pressure forces the government to keep in place laws that criminalize sex work and sexual intercourse between men. Public health workers are therefore faced with a real challenge. They need to help keep public health in check but at the same time they cannot give the impression they are breaking the law or supporting those who do so. As a result, she and her colleagues often worked by night to educate and sensitize MSM and sex workers concerning healthy living. And night after night she and her colleagues had to run from the police, because they dare not be caught with clients or patients who are assumed to be trading in sex. Here is an example of a woman of faith, working with the government, but having a real conflict in living out what it means to say God cares for people.

Third, she is not only a person of faith and a staff member of the Ministry of Health: she also lives in Jamaica. In any church congregation, it is likely that an average of 80 percent will express disapproval of MSM and people who engage in sex work. This is the national average. So with that said, we must ask how Christians, like this nurse, should respond to the needs of those who engage in such lifestyles. These are key populations in the struggle against HIV. Ignoring their existence would have implications for the entire population. "Stop what you are doing," we could say. But that is to be blind to the human stories that lie behind decisions to adopt such life styles. Some therefore accept, understand, and sympathize with these vulnerable, stigmatized people. But within the church there are many who will quote the book of Leviticus and Paul's letter to the Romans as evidence for condemning such practices. These people may speak apocalyptically of our challenging times, signalling the advent of "the last days," when we should be punished with devastation and destruction.

Implications for the church in the Caribbean

As a church, we must ask the question: In such contexts, how are we to proclaim the message that God cares for all God's people?

For the church in the Caribbean, responding to HIV and AIDS has proved a challenge to our understanding of pastoral care and of ethics. As practical theologian Stephen Pattison says, "Pastoral care which takes the social and political dimensions of human existence seriously should probably adopt a bias to the poor in the pastoral situation."[2] A church of and for the poor is required to embrace a social and political stance that indicates that God cares for people. Here in the Caribbean, the poorest are those living with, affected by, or vulnerable to HIV and AIDS. We have therefore proclaimed God's care for all by adopting a social and political stance that points to God's love and care for people, especially those who are the poorest and most vulnerable. As a result, although high levels of stigma and discrimination still pose challenges for the practice of pastoral care, HIV is gradually coming to be accepted as a chronic illness.

Ethically, then, the church in the Caribbean and other religious groups have taken up the challenge to value the lives of all people. Theologian John Wilkinson recommends a principle-based approach to the practice of Christian ethics. Loving your neighbour as yourself, he says, is a golden rule. Value people for who they are and not what others think they ought to be, he urges.[3]

It is undeniably difficult to affirm God's care for people in such context, but we have found that by practising those golden rules it is possible to love and value people like Andrew even when members of their family abandon them.

In the final analysis two things are critical if religious institutions are to successfully challenge the HIV epidemic in the Caribbean. The first is effective leadership designed to combat the kinds of actions and attitudes displayed by the church member mentioned in my opening paragraphs. The second is a combined pastoral and ethical stance that will focus on God's care for all people. This stance must be accompanied by policies and programmes that affirm people's value, irrespective of age, gender, ethnicity, sexual orientation, and religious persuasion. Every one of us is made in the image of God. People like Andrew deserve respect and love.

Question for discussion

• What advice would you give to the woman nurse whose dilemmas are described in the second section of this essay?

Part Three

Some Theological Entry Points

What does the Lord ask of you? To act justly, to love mercy
and to walk humbly with your God.
– Micah 6:8

In Part One we explored some critical issues that are regularly
encountered in faith-aware discourses on HIV, AIDS, and human rights. In
Part Two we met men and women, from all over the world, whose personal
experience and ministry have given them vivid insights into the struggles
involved in bringing human rights principles to bear on individual political,
cultural, and social contexts, particularly in responding to HIV and AIDS.

In Part Three, we have invited three Christian theologians, working with
the experiences that came out of the discussions that led to this book, to share
their reflections on what, for them, have been the most helpful theological
entry points to this sometimes-difficult discussion. All of them have long experience of working at the cutting edge of Christian responses to HIV and AIDS,
and of the potential of theological and scriptural beliefs to support or to undermine effective responses to HIV and AIDS. It should be stressed, therefore,
that none of them believes that they have the last word. On the contrary, it
is our hope that these thoughts will inspire you, our readers, to initiate such
discussions in your own groups and in relation to your own contexts. As with
previous chapters, we have suggested some questions you might like to work
with: but you are just as likely to have your own.

Chapter 17

The Redemption of God's Good Gift of Sexuality

Michael Schuenemeyer

HIV, AIDS and human sexuality

In the beginning, say the early chapters of Genesis, God looked on everything God had created and declared that it was not merely "good," it was *very* good." And that included the creation of human sexuality, which is just as important as every other part of creation that God declared "very good." In other words, when God proclaimed all of creation very good, God was proclaiming human sexuality very good, as well. This good gift of sexuality is something God bestows on every person, created as we all are in God's image. To be a whole person, therefore, is to be a sexual person, at whatever age, whether abstinent or sexually active, married, partnered or single, able-bodied or differently-abled. From inside the womb to the time we are born until the time we die, we are sexual beings.

This is a fundamentally important baseline for any reflection on HIV, AIDS, and human rights, mainly because public attitudes to the epidemic have been so closely bound up with people's attitudes to sex, sexuality, and sexual behaviour; this association which is one of the factors that have led to people living with HIV or AIDS being viewed as somehow less than human, or entitled to fewer rights than others. But human sexuality is more than engaging in sexual behaviour. What it means is that all people, in all their diversities, have feelings, desires, sensations, and the need for relationships of mutual care, trust, and intimacy. That is a healthy, holy, positive, good, and integral part of each and every human person.

Furthermore, the good gift of sexuality is as diverse as every other gift that God has bestowed on God's children. Every person, as a child of God, is endowed by God with worth and dignity that human judgment cannot set aside. This is a fundamental, gospel value that undergirds the foundations of Christian community, as well all human rights.

Throughout the history of Christianity, though, positive messages about sexuality have – regrettably – been the exception. From the legacy of the ancient Jewish purity codes to St Augustine, from the Puritans to the Victorians, sexuality has too often been viewed as evil and sexual behaviour as sinful. Even within bonds of marriage, sex has been considered a sin, necessary for the sake of having children, but a sin nonetheless. This has led to a silence surrounding sexual matters, which cedes the ground to the powers and principalities that exploit human sexuality for the sake of greed and create vulnerabilities to abusive and predatory practices.

In relation to HIV and AIDS, the negative messages emerging from Christian and other religious traditions have heaped shame, guilt, and self-loathing on God's children, leading sometimes to violence and death perpetrated in the name of Christ. In many cultures, such messages have created fear, stigma, and discrimination, jeopardizing the health and wholeness of whole populations. The legacy of human rights abuses and atrocities stands as a damning indictment against a significant portion of the Christian tradition. The HIV pandemic has been and continues to be a tragic testament to these realities.

This isn't to say that churches are doing nothing: many are doing a great deal. Nevertheless, the overall trend has been to be silent, if not resistant, to sexuality education, especially in terms of sexual orientation and gender identity, barrier methods of contraception, and other areas of sexual and reproductive health. The church becomes complicit in the progression of the epidemic when it fails to break the silence about sexuality and HIV: a failure that a former UNAIDS ambassador has termed "murder by complacency." For example, Rev. Dr Kapya Kaomo documents the fomenting of anti-gay sentiment in Uganda and other countries, influenced by some evangelical Christian groups in the US.[1] Again, the church has not been able to respond effectively to gender-based violence when it is stuck, as it often is, in a patriarchal system that exploits women. None of this is new. But the HIV epidemic has thrown a spotlight on attitudes and practices that have been around for centuries by exploiting the vulnerabilities and abuses they create.

Archbishop Desmond Tutu has spoken about this with passion. "Silence kills, stigma kills," he says. "We should not want those living with HIV to be the modern equivalent of the biblical leper who had to carry a bell and a sign saying 'I am unclean.'"[2] It is the ethical and moral duty of faith communities and religious leaders to break the silence and negativity that surrounds this epidemic, and to transform the faith conversation from sex-negative to sex-positive. For the sake of the whole human family, we must redeem the good gift of human sexuality. In this task we are called, as faith communities, to build and strengthen our capacities to create safe spaces, show grace in relation to difference, welcome different theological perspectives, and take action to support and uphold the human rights of all people, including those of different sexes, sexual orientations, gender identities, and expressions.

To change the conversation in this way, we begin, first, by engaging a positive rubric for biblical interpretation, grounded in redemptive grace, love and justice; and second, by cultivating a culture in our churches that embraces faith-based, age-appropriate, comprehensive sexuality education.

Engaging a positive rubric for biblical interpretation

In 2005, in the US, the United Church of Christ brought together about 150 clergy of colour to discuss issues of theology and human sexuality. Old Testament scholar Dr Randall Bailey led into the opening lecture and discussion by asking the participants if they had enjoyed the buffet the night before, where the main course was pork ribs and shrimp. There was enthusiastic applause. He then opened the scriptures at the book of Leviticus and read out the prohibitions against eating pork and shellfish. The text is unambiguous. Eating pork or shellfish is an abomination against God. And yet here was his audience using some abomination texts to condemn others' behaviour, but refusing to apply abomination texts that condemned their own. His point was that double standards exist ("hypocrisy," Jesus would have called it). In dealing with sacred texts, no matter where we stand on the "contextual" versus "literal" interpretation spectrum, it is critical to recognize and avoid the use of such double standards.

It is equally important to be discerning about the rubric we will employ in understanding the meaning of the text. Whether we are conscious of it or not, each of us has a lens through which we engage with and derive meaning from scripture. So for Christians, as disciples of Jesus, it is helpful to look at how Jesus approached scripture. It doesn't take long to realize that Jesus did not employ a literal approach to the Torah, his sacred text. "You have heard it said…, but I tell you" (Matt. 5:21ff) are *not* the words of a literalist. Jesus practised and invited a contextual approach. The key to our discernment is what we witness and experience of the Spirit.

For example, John the Baptist sent his disciples to ask Jesus if he was the one to come or should they look for another. "Go," said Jesus, "and tell John what you have seen and heard: the blind receive their sight, the lame walk, the lepers are cleansed, the deaf hear, the dead are raised, the poor have good news brought to them. And blessed is anyone who takes no offense at me" (Luke 7:19-23). The scriptures teach us to be discerning about what the Holy Spirit is up to and to recognize the abundance of God's blessing in our relationships. Jesus said, "I have come that you may have life, and have it abundantly" (John 10:10). Martin Luther King, Jr said, "The moral arc of the universe is long but it bends towards justice," to which Old Testament scholar Walter Brueggemann adds, "and the moral arc of the Gospel bends toward inclusion."[3]

This was certainly true of the early Christian church. Acts records the amazing diversity of people who experienced the power of the Holy Spirit at Pentecost (Acts 2). Through his encounter with the Ethiopian eunuch, Phillip experiences the presence of the Holy Spirit and offers him the sacrament of baptism (Acts 8:27ff). Peter, having received a vision of inclusion, accepts the invitation to stay with the household of Cornelius, which leads to the baptism of the whole household (Acts 10). These were gentiles, about whom the Hebrew scriptures stated clearly that they were not to be included.

Yet the grace of God prevailed. The Bible is replete with such stories of how the supposedly unclean, unacceptable, untouchable, excluded, marginalized ones are reconciled and healed, how they experience the grace of God and frequently become God's chosen leaders. Our task as a Christian community, rooted in our scriptures, is to seek out the ways in which the God of love, peace, and justice is present in our lives and in our world, including the life-giving ways God is present in our understanding and experience of this good gift of sexuality.

Embracing faith-based, age-appropriate, comprehensive sexuality education

There can be little doubt that the attitudes of Christian traditions and teachings have, too often, done more to perpetuate vulnerability, marginalization, stigma, and discrimination than to support convictions of the wholeness and healthiness of human sexuality. It doesn't have to be this way. Especially in a time of HIV and AIDS, people need accurate, non-judgmental information about the different facets of sexuality. It is normal that expressions of sexuality should vary according to one's age, stage of human development, knowledge, cultural context, life circumstances, and values: including faith values. This is a significant reason why life-span, age-appropriate, comprehensive sexuality education needs to be an integral part of each person's development and formation at every stage of life.

If we really believe that sexuality is a good gift that comes from God, then church is not only an appropriate place for sexuality education like this, but it should be the ideal place for it. As in other aspects of culture, sexuality, sexual expectations, and sexuality education are dependent on common values shared across the community. God's call to us to be human and the redemption of God's healthy, holy, good gift of sexuality are dependent on the church acquiring the competencies and skills necessary to provide a safe environment in which the whole community can learn.

So how can the church become a grace-filled place where people can learn about the complexities of human sexuality, receive accurate information, develop and clarify their faith values, and gain the experience and skills needed to live their values in the real world of their day-to-day experience?

Our Whole Lives is a faith-based, life-span, age-appropriate, comprehensive sexuality education curriculum developed through a partnership of the United Church of Christ (UCC) and the Unitarian Universalist Association and grounded in the values of self-worth, sexual health, responsibility, justice, and inclusion. The following principles, it suggests, should support an understanding of the interconnectedness of sexuality and spirituality:

Sexuality is a God-given gift.
The purposes of sexuality are to enhance human wholeness and fulfilment; to express love, commitment, delight, and pleasure; to bring new life into the world; and to give glory to God.
When making decisions about sexuality, the primary goal is God's call to love and justice as revealed in both Testaments.
From a biblical perspective, sexuality is intended to express mutuality, love, and justice. In judging whether behaviour is ethical or unethical, the norms of mutuality, love, and justice are the central criteria.

From a biblical perspective, sexuality is distorted by unethical behaviours, attitudes, and systems that foster violence, exploitation, infidelity, assertion of power, and the treatment of persons as objects.

In developing a just sexual morality, we need to avoid double standards.

A responsible and mature sexual ethic respects the moral agency of every person.

The church, at all levels, ought to be a context for discussion about human sexuality.

The church ought to encourage and support advocacy with those who are sexually oppressed or are victims of sexual violence and abuse. The church can and must have a role in defining and implementing public policy.

—*Our Whole Lives*

Before we rush to judgment in relation to people living with or affected by HIV or AIDS, we should remember that the message which most clearly resonates throughout the Gospel is the message of love and grace. More than anything else about the way of Jesus, permeating his life and ministry is his consistent outreach to the disadvantaged and disenfranchised. He repeatedly went against the conventions of the culture and religious authorities of his time. He regularly addressed judgmental attitudes and actions that created vulnerabilities and marginalized people. Jesus never turned anyone away, and the only ones he treated with contempt were religious authorities who did nothing to address the injustices in their midst and which they helped to perpetuate through their actions or complacency.

So to sum up: if we want our churches to be true game-changers in global and local responses to HIV and AIDS, we need to honour the worth and dignity of every person as a child of God; to develop a positive, grace-filled rubric for interpreting scripture grounded in love and justice; and to cultivate a culture for faith-based, life-span, age-appropriate comprehensive sexuality education. This will not only redeem God's good gift of human sexuality, it will play a significant role in ending the HIV epidemic. In the words of the *Our Whole Lives* curriculum, the entire community benefits, is blessed, and may become a more just and loving place for everyone as together we learn to sing the music of positive, healthy, holy sexuality.

Publication mentioned in this text

Our Whole Lives is a faith-based, life-span, age-appropriate, comprehensive sexuality education curriculum developed through a partnership of the United Church of Christ (UCC) and the Unitarian Universalist Association. It may be accessed via: www.ucc.org/owl

Questions for discussion

Reflecting on the statement, "Our task as a Christian community, rooted in our scriptures, is to seek out the ways in which the God of love, peace and justice is present in our lives and in our world, including the life-giving ways God is present in our understanding and experience of this good gift of sexuality":

- Is this indeed the task of a Christian community?
- In what ways do our own community succeed in carrying it out?
- What might help us to do better?

Chapter 18

The Image of God: Recognizing God within Key Populations

Ijeoma Ajibade

Understanding the *Imago Dei*

The *imago Dei* is the Latin term for the "image of God": a phrase that is found within the biblical account of creation where God speaks about "making humankind in our own image" (Gen. 1:26-27). *Imago Dei* implies a mandate of power and responsibility, given by God to human beings, to exercise in relation to both human and non-human creation. So God created human beings to be his representatives on earth, and we are to manage the earth for the welfare of all. In this, God shows a particular concern for the welfare of humanity, as distinct from the rest of creation. The idea of *imago Dei* points to the special qualities of human nature that allow God to be made manifest in human beings, and it also gives us a strong theological sense of having a shared humanity: shared, that is, with each other and with the God in whose image we are made. This makes it a powerful image in any theological reflection on HIV and AIDS.

The HIV pandemic and key populations: Exclusion, invisibility and vulnerability

> What I found with all of these faith-based churches was that as soon as I mentioned that I was an active drug user I was quickly asked to step down from the membership, excommunicated and informed that I was back slider, was denied partaking in Holy Communion, was told that I did not truly have salvation. (Mags Maher, UK)[1]

In many ways it has been easy for the church to ignore the pandemic, because it predominantly affects people whose lives may not accord with the ethical and moral beliefs of its members. These include men who have sex with men, sex workers, intravenous drug users, and people who are poor and unable to access health care. These groups of people can be described as "key populations." They are people who are excluded from mainstream societies because they are disapproved of. This exclusion means that they are invisible to the people who develop policies within our societies; and ultimately, then, their needs (including health, social, educational, and economic) are often overlooked. This, in turn, makes these populations vulnerable to all kinds of ill health and social disadvantage.

The *imago Dei*, though, wipes away excuses and inaction and actually places a responsibility on the church not to forget or ignore key populations.

> A sex worker is a sister, a cousin, an auntie and a mother to members of your community. She is a member of your community! (Peninah Mwangi, Kenya).

Other writers in this publication have demonstrated ways in which the HIV pandemic exposes the fault lines of our societies. For example, poverty, social marginalization, and discrimination have enabled the virus to flourish in our world today, largely because the people who are most affected are the very people that societies all over the world ignore. Despite this, it has become possible to envisage an AIDS-free future. The vision of the global AIDS movement is to have zero new HIV infections, zero discrimination, and zero AIDS-related deaths. As the pandemic enters its fourth decade, though, we realize that this vision will only be achieved if country governments continue to sustain their efforts in both treatment and prevention, and if they invest the necessary financial resources. In many countries today, death from AIDS is no longer inevitable, and some countries are re-classifying AIDS as a "critical" (as opposed to a "terminal") illness. So we are at a tipping point, needing a fresh new wave of mobilization that calls people to review the history of the pandemic. Responding to current challenges must involve a new younger generation that is willing to continue with activism and pressure, not just on governments but on all sectors of society, including faith communities and the church.

> The voices of the people in the periphery, mostly the key population, are not heard because societies including the church consider them as the worst sinners. Yet . . . Jesus loved and embraced the prostitute in John 18:1-8, and unlike the leaders of the day, Jesus broke all barriers and related with the woman in a dignifying manner. (Dr Beatrice Okyere-Manu, South Africa)

The church and HIV

Looking back, we have to admit that churches have not always responded as they should to key populations. Much of our history, at the beginning of the pandemic, was shameful. In the early 1980s in the US and Europe, when HIV and AIDS first appeared in the gay communities, the initial response from some churches was a mixture of confusion and condemnation. Some churches saw HIV and AIDS as a form of divine judgment, particularly against homosexuals. Botswanan biblical scholar Musa Dube speaks of the Bible being used to support this stance, referring to Old Testament narratives of God using illness and disease as a means of punishing disobedience.

But it was not just religious groups that were acting this way. Across the world, responses to HIV and AIDS were driven by fear, resulting in stigma and discrimination that continues today in many forms. Epidemiologists point out that this initial response was a normal stage in the human struggle to come to terms with a new and frightening disease. For the church, though, it was a missed opportunity to demonstrate the compassion of Christ, a missed opportunity to recognize the *imago Dei* in our key populations, and therefore a missed opportunity to address their exclusion, invisibility, and vulnerability.

> I have never been so creative in planning ways to kill myself. When I had an adverse reaction to Nevirapine during my ARV trial, I wished the high fever would finally kill me. When I tried to regain some hope about life, I applied for an international scholarship. I declared my HIV status and thought that it would be an advantage, as they stated preferential option for people with disabilities. They rejected my application. Maybe it was my new drug, Efavirenz,

but for me HIV killed my dreams, and I wished that I had thrown myself in front of a truck. (Marcus, Philippines)

Thankfully in many places the attitude of churches has changed and many are leading responses to HIV that are informed, understanding, and compassionate. All over the world we now have Christian ministries devoted to the care and support of people living with HIV. We also have major faith-based development agencies at the forefront of the HIV response. There are all kinds of publications and resources available to help churches understand how to respond to HIV within their local contexts and globally. But has the church gone far enough? There is still much more it can do in order to secure this vision of an AIDS-free future. Recognizing the *imago Dei* in our key populations will give the church a new vision and impetus to become further involved in HIV and to engage with the people who are most affected.

Stigma against key populations can be overcome if the highest values of the faith are stressed, namely, love and compassion, hope and health. (Peninah Mwangi, Kenya)

The *imago Dei*

Imago Dei theology points us toward various different ways humanity is to be distinguished from non-human creation. Bringing these separate aspects together and reading them holistically can help deepen our understanding of what it means to be created "in the image of God."

Theologian Colin Gunton points to five main strands in *imago Dei* theology, namely "mind and reason," "freedom," "co-creation," "relationship," and "dominion." These strands come together in our theological reflection on HIV and AIDS. From the medieval to the early modern period, it was believed that the *imago Dei* was a product of the human mind, and of the human capacity for reason. But in emphasizing reason alone and neglecting the body, this view fails to take account of the fact that human beings are more than just intellect. A more modern theological understanding of *imago Dei* emphasizes its relevance to human freedom. God acts freely, therefore humans have the same capacity to act freely and be self-determining. It is this capacity that shows that humans are made in the image of God.

Other understandings focus on God as Creator. Since God creates, humans must see themselves as co-creators: a theme developed by Pope John

Paul ll in *Laborem Exercens (On Human Work)*. They do this in relationship with each other, with God, and with non-human creation, thus emphasizing the theme of relationship, which itself derives from a trinitarian understanding of the nature of God. So just as there is relationship within the nature of God between Father, Son, and Holy Spirit, humans are created to be part of that relationship. In the Genesis account, God gives human beings dominion over creation (Gen. 1:26). But this does not mean humanity is given permission to exploit or dominate. Colin Gunton defines dominion as "a responsibility under God for the proper perfecting of created things."[2] The kind of dominion we are talking about takes account of the fact that we exist in relation to others and to non-human creation.

Bringing these themes together provides us with a basic understanding of what it means to be made in the image of God. Taken together with those other great themes of Trinity and of creation, a deeper meaning emerges and guidance becomes available to help us know how we should live. Specifically, it places responsibility on the church not to stand back from key populations but to find a way to engage with the marginalized people of this world, in the knowledge that everything we believe about the *imago Dei* for ourselves is also true of others, whoever they may be.

> Deconstructing our messages may mean revisiting the discourse of the theology of human beings made in the image of God. And not to see them through what they do but as people who are loved and created in the image of God and that their "being" is more important to God. (Beatrice Okyere-Manu, South Africa)

> It was a dead end for me then. That is until I found a faith-based support group for people living with HIV in the Philippines. With every seeker I met at the meetings, I found someone who shared the same wounds of being pushed to the margins because of who they are. I have been with people who have been mired in the very same dark holes of self-hatred because of what their families and faith communities have made them believe all this while. I have seen that all of them have come to find an affirmation that God loves them and there is nothing at all to fix, for we were never broken to begin with. (Marcus, Philippines)

Engaging key populations

To sum up: the *imago Dei* reminds us that we all bear the imprint of God. In this way it challenges our tendency to exclude or marginalize others. If God is present in men who have sex with men, sex workers, intravenous drug users, people who are poor, and other key populations, then to ignore or to marginalize them is to ignore or marginalize God.

> In the eyes of the church and society drug users are generally often seen as the scourge of society, and are a marginalized group on the very fringes of society without a voice. Many drug users who have a faith and belief in God are often unable to approach their church leaders and disclose their drug use for fear of further judgment, discrimination, and marginalization. (Mags Maher, UK)

Further, many of our key populations have a profound religious faith:

> A study carried out by BHESP in Thika town (Kenya) shows that 80 percent of sex workers are Christians. Sixty percent of sex workers in Thika attend church regularly, and twenty percent tithe. Eight percent of sex workers with children have had them baptized in church. (Peninah Mwangi, Kenya)

The *imago Dei* implies that every human being has dignity. We must learn how to relate to those people who are not the same as us. When we see our communities divided by race, gender, sexual orientation, class and age, we should remember that we are – all of us – created in the image of God; and we should have the confidence to produce reasoned arguments for challenging societal attitudes and facing up to the prejudice that lies within us all. It is part of the mission of the church and part of our prophetic witness to live in such a way that we influence all spheres of life. Other people bear the imprint of God even when we feel they don't adhere to our standards.

This will not just develop support for people living with HIV within their own communities. It could also, by raising awareness about HIV, assist with the implementation of prevention strategies. Church leaders will then enter into dialogue with people from key populations and we will begin to live the theology of the *imago Dei*, in the confidence that God loves us and blesses us as humanity. Thus we will come to a place where we begin to see the image of God in others, an image that binds us together in our humanity even when we choose to ignore or marginalize it.

I am now part of a programme that is currently working on a positive policy environment on sexuality. I hope to work with our local churches on appropriate interventions to address the access to HIV prevention, testing, and treatment services for the key populations most vulnerable to HIV – men who have sex with men, people in prison, people who inject drugs, sex workers, and transgender people. (Marcus, Philippines)

Resources

Bonhoeffer, Dietrich. *Creation and Temptation* (SCM Press London, 1966).

Fowler, Norman. *AIDS: Don't Die of Prejudice* (Biteback Publishing, 2014).

Gunton, Colin E. *The Christian Faith, an Introduction to Christian Doctrine* (Blackwell Publishing Oxford, 2002).

Gunton, Colin E. *The One, The Three and The Many. God Creation and the Culture of Modernity* (Cambridge University Press, 1993).

Gunton, Colin E. *The Promise of Trinitarian Theology* (T&T Clark Edinburgh, 1991).

Gunton, Colin E. *The Triune Creator: A Historical and Systematic Study* (Edinburgh: Edinburgh University Press, 1998).

Musa, Dube, W. *HIV/AIDS and the Curriculum* (WCC Publications, Geneva, 2003).

Questions for discussion

- How does the idea of *imago Dei* affect your image of yourself? How does it affect your image of those most marginalized in society?

- Does your own church community include individuals who are particularly vulnerable? Why are they vulnerable? How might the idea of *imago Dei* affect the way they are included in the community?

Chapter 19

Gender Inequality and Human Rights: A Prophetic Trinitarian Anthropology

Nontando Hadebe

Trinity, gender, and rights

Trinitarian theology provides an illuminating lens for approaching the relationship between gender inequality and human rights, HIV, and AIDS. As a theoretical construct, it suggests that Christian understandings of the Trinity – Father, Son and Holy Spirit – provide a valuable framework for understanding the importance of the wider social context in human experience: a social context that must be taken seriously in any discussion of individual cases of human rights. This challenges popular understandings that view HIV and AIDS as God's punishment for sexual immorality, as it also challenges the tendency of many Christians to adopt stigmatizing and judgmental attitudes toward people living with HIV and AIDS.

Compare, for example, two common approaches to HIV and AIDS. I shall call them "morality only" and "evidence-based human rights." In the "morality only" approach, people living with HIV and AIDS are judged to have acquired the infection through sexual immorality and therefore "deserve" to suffer. In contrast, the "evidence-based human rights" approach takes into account those wider social factors (culture, religion, gender, biology, poverty, and so on) that create a context of vulnerability to HIV infection. For example, poverty drives some women to engage in sex work, and some cultural norms encourage men to have multiple partners: both factors contributing to a context of vulnerability to HIV infection.

The role of contextual human experience also separates two approaches to theology. Contextual theologian Stephen Bevans describes these as the "classical" and the "contextual." Classical approaches to moral and theological judgments do not take account of human experience. Contextual approaches, on the other hand, seek to engage with all aspects of human experience, opening the way to a relationship between trinitarian theology, gender, and justice.

In this chapter, therefore, I am taking a contextual approach to the challenges of HIV and AIDS in Southern Africa. In particular, I want to address a key driver of the epidemic in this region, namely gender, which I am defining, here, as "the social constructions that are associated with biological sexual difference, determining what it means to be female or male in our society."

But what has this to do with the Holy Trinity?

A central belief of Christianity is that all human beings are created in the image of God. This Christian God is Trinity: and that means God is a loving communion of three different persons (Father, Son, and Holy Spirit), whose "being-in-relation" is revealed in liberating actions toward human beings. So the idea of relationship is at the heart of our understanding of the nature of God. This belief has particular implications for the way we view relationships and the importance we attach to social and economic contexts. Under the reign of this trinitarian God, the characteristics of difference, equality, communion, unity, inter-relatedness, interdependence, and justice become part of our understanding of what it is to be human. As an African, I find it interesting to note how closely these understandings align with our traditional beliefs about the human person as related and in community.

We have already noted that gender roles, in the context of HIV and AIDS, are a contributing factor to vulnerability. The question that trinitarian theology needs to answer is the following: "Can this theology lead us toward a prophetic Christian anthropology that confronts and transforms gender from being a source of vulnerability to being an alternative liberative paradigm of human persons?" I believe that trinitarian theology, despite its dominant male representation of God, does have the resources to open the way to a view of Christian community where difference, equality, community, and justice coexist.

Theology and context

The observations in this next section highlight two studies from KwaZulu Natal (one by the KZN Christian Council, and one by PACSA, the Pietermaritzburg Agency for Community Social Action), and are followed by some comments from the writings of the late Dr Jonathan Mann, late director of the global AIDS program of the World Health Organization (WHO).

Throughout the PACSA study[1] we encounter the view that immoral lifestyles are the root causes of HIV and AIDS. The KwaZulu-Natal Christian Council study[2] also notes that the church's view of HIV and AIDS is focused on sexual behaviour, and that this association between HIV and moral behaviour resulted in judgmental and stigmatizing attitudes toward people living with HIV or AIDS. When respondents living with HIV said they longed for safe spaces to tell their stories, it was essentially a cry for the church to re-examine its judgmental and stigmatizing attitudes in the light of contextual human experience.

As director of WHO's AIDS program, Jonathan Mann pioneered the movement for a more rights-based approach to HIV and AIDS. He states:

> In each society those people who before HIV and AIDS arrived were marginalized, stigmatized and discriminated against become over time those at highest risk of HIV infection. . . . A human rights based approach provides a common vocabulary for describing the commonalities that underlie the specific situations of vulnerable people around the world and clarity about the necessary direction of health-promoting change.[3]

Following this, a human rights-based approach was urged in all of the UN's agencies and member states, including all of the countries in Southern Africa. In particular, in any prevention programme it became good practice to promote gender equality, address gender norms that created vulnerability for women and girls, and involve men in this effort. Thus, vulnerability to HIV infection came to be seen as related to the wider social contexts of injustice, and the pursuit of human rights becomes an essential part of the prevention strategy.

It may be helpful, here, to distinguish between classical and contextual ways of doing theology. The work of contextual theologian Stephen Bevans, mentioned above, sets out the distinction especially clearly. Classical theology, he says, "conceived theology as a kind of objective science of faith. It was understood as a reflection in faith on . . . scripture and tradition, the content of which has not and never will be changed, and is above culture and historically conditioned expression."[4] Contextual theology, though, recognizes another source of theological understanding, in the form of recent human experience. "Theology that is contextual," says Bevans, "realizes that culture, history, contemporary thought forms and so forth are to be considered, along with scripture and tradition, as valid sources for theological expression."

But how does this relate to gender?

Gender in the context of HIV and AIDS in Southern Africa

Gender is a key driver of the epidemic in Southern Africa, its impact evident in the failure of prevention efforts with women and girls. An example of this is the widely applied ABC method (A - Abstain from sexual activities; B - Be faithful to a single sexual partner or spouse; or C - condoms to be used in every sexual intercourse.) For the majority of women and girls in Southern Africa, these rules of thumb are quite unrealistic, failing, as the UNAIDS report puts it, to "take into account the gender and other inequalities that shape people's behaviours and limit their choices."[5]

Men's assumptions are generally defined by corresponding cultural convictions, leading men to believe that masculinity requires them to seek multiple partnerships, exercise power over women, and demonstrate economic success: all of which create vulnerabilities for men. Further research has shown that failure to fulfil these masculinity ideals is a contributing factor to the increase in male sexual violence against women, while other writers have observed that sexual violence and masculinity are themselves related to broader political and economic changes, such as colonialism, job losses, and poverty. We see this when young men find themselves prevented by poverty from paying bride wealth, taking wives, fathering children, or establishing their own homesteads.

The preservation of culture is often given as a reason for denying women's rights. Theologian Musimbi Kanyoro believes that "all questions regarding the welfare and status of women in Africa are explainable within the framework of culture."[6] But culture is far from being a stable, easily recognizable, static, and unchallengeable entity. Instead of using culture as a justification for human rights violations, Kanyoro says, we should rather be asking (a) whose interests are served by traditions and customs that control women's autonomy, sexuality, production, and reproduction?" and (b) "who is defining culture?" It is not that culture should be ignored: but it should not be uncritically accepted either.

Gender and Trinity

In claiming that trinitarian theology challenges Christian beliefs about the nature of God, it is hardly necessary to point out that one of those beliefs is that God is male. The idea of God-as-Father together with associated use of the language of fatherhood have supported male domination in the church and society and given powerful support to the oppression of women.

In practice, though, the images of Father presented by Jesus critiqued and destabilized patriarchy. Examples include Jesus' use of female images for God in stories like the woman searching for her lost coin (Luke 15:8-10) and in the incorporation of women in the circle of disciples following Jesus (Luke 8:1-2).

However, in recent years, the theological links between patriarchy, inequality, and subordination of women have encountered challenges from liberation and feminist theologians, and also from the movement to explore social models of the Trinity. Emphasizing the absolute importance of context, the proponents of Social Models of Trinity define the human person as inescapably relational, concrete, and communitarian. This description aligns with African communitarian beliefs on the human person as communal and related: beliefs that are reflected in the saying "*umuntu ngumuntu ngabantu*" ("a person is a person through others").[7]

Addressing inequality: A radical prophetic-pastoral trinitarian anthropology

In the context of HIV and AIDS, gender analysis has demonstrated the processes by which cultural and religious norms support gender-based vulnerabilities to HIV infection that affect both women and men. For Christianity, then, the challenge is to develop an alternative gender paradigm that does not eliminate differences but addresses inequality.

The World Health Organization, in its publication *Gender, Women and Health*, defines gender difference as "the distinctive roles and behaviors of men and women in a given culture dictated by that culture's gender norms and values." Gender inequality, it is said, results from "differences between men and women which systematically empower one group to the detriment of the other. . . . The gender picture in any given time and place can be one of the major obstacles - sometimes the single most important obstacle – standing between men and women and the achievement of well-being."[8]

The HIV pandemic has been a source of revelation on the impact of gender inequality on the wellbeing of both women and men. The core challenge then becomes not how to iron out differences, nor to use it as an excuse for one group's supremacy, but to hold together differences and equality within a community. For such a relationship, the Trinity provides a powerful model. As Leonardo Boff noted,

> In the Trinity there is no domination by one side, but convergence of the Three in mutual acceptance and giving. They are different but none is greater or lesser, before or after. Therefore a society that takes its inspiration from Trinitarian communion cannot tolerate class differences, dominations based on power (economic, sexual or ideological) that subjects those who are different to those who exercise that power and marginalizes the former from the latter.[9]

A Christian anthropology based on trinitarian theology is therefore radical and prophetic, defining the human person in terms of difference, equality, community, inter-dependence, and relatedness. Within this paradigm, as Boff says, there is no room for injustice in any form. Thus the wider social factors that create vulnerability to HIV infection are challenged as an integral part of efforts to eliminate the epidemic and produce a society in which such vulnerabilities are countered.

Conclusion

This paper has appropriated a central belief of Christianity, namely the Trinity, to address the challenges of HIV and AIDS that have devastated lives, communities, and nations. It has demonstrated how approaches to HIV and approaches to Christian theology have come together to challenge some Christians responses to PLHIV. This has been especially true in relation to the role of faith in responding to contextual challenges. When it proclaims justice, faith first responds to context and then applies Christian resources to that response.

The witness of scripture is that God is not indifferent or passive in the face of human suffering. Hence we hear the call to live out the image of God in accordance with the passion for justice and liberation that defines God. To be fully human is to have a God-like passion for justice, and to promote communities of difference, equality, mutuality, and love. All of that reflects fundamental African beliefs about the human person. In this way, trinitarian anthropology, as a response to gender challenges in the context of HIV and AIDS in Southern Africa, brings together the ideals of culture, human rights, and Christianity in service to communities.

Resources

Boff, Leonardo. *Trinity and Society*, translated from the Portuguese by Paul Burns. Oregon: Wipf & Stock Publishers, 1998.

Johnson, Elizabeth. *She Who Is: The Mystery of God in Feminist Theological Discourse*. New York: CrossRoads, 1992.

Kanyoro, Musimbi. *Introducing Feminist Cultural Hermeneutics: An African Perspective*. London: Sheffield Academic Press.

O'Collins, Gerald. *The Tripersonal God: Understanding and Interpreting the Trinity*. New York: Paulist Press, 1999.

Questions for discussion

- God is Trinity, therefore God is "inescapably relational and communitarian," says this writer. Where do you find these relational, trinitarian characteristics in your own society or community? With what other values might they come into conflict?

- How does your church or Christian community handle difference? Does it deal with some kinds of difference more successfully than others? In what contexts might difference lead to actual discrimination, and can this ever be justified?

- In your everyday life, do you encounter situations where gender inequality has resulted in human rights being overlooked? How might a person justify the denial of human rights on grounds of gender?

Epilogue

Gillian Paterson

> They will not leave within you one stone upon another,
> because you did not recognize the time of your visitation
> from God.
> —Luke 19:44b

A *Kairos* moment

Kairos is a Greek word that means "an opportune moment," or a "passing instant when an opening appears which must be driven through if success is to be achieved." In the 1980s, churches in South Africa believed they were facing just such a "*Kairos* moment" in the struggle against apartheid, and a group of theologians came together to develop what came to be known as *The Kairos Document*. From this small beginning grew a movement that helped to change the face of South Africa, offering new ways of thinking about present realities and delivering a powerful theological judgment on the apartheid state and its denial to its citizens of freedom, justice, and human dignity.

The Kairos Document identified three theological "systems" that were proving to be positioning factors in South Africa's political struggles at that time. It is important to note that Christians were vocal in all three, with Christian scriptures being quoted as grounds for justifying the three widely differing positions they represented. First, the document critiqued "State Theology": in this case, the claim that the cultural, political, and traditional status quo is sanctified by God, even if it is demonstrably harmful to a large proportion of the population. Next it commented on what it termed "Church Theology," meaning the actions and statements of the majority of mainstream churches. Church Theology, it said, attempts a critique of the status quo, but "its criticism is superficial . . . because . . . it relies on a few stock ideas from Christian tradition and then uncritically accepts them and applies them to our situation."[1]

Finally, there was a third option, which the *Kairos* theologians called "Prophetic Theology." Prophetic theology had a strong emphasis on justice. It prioritized experiences of suffering and oppression. And it insisted on the value of social, political and economic analysis in interpreting the "signs of the times." A prophetic theology will first address what is true, said the *Kairos* theologians, and then it will call for action. It will place a great emphasis on hope, it will be deeply spiritual, it will denounce sin and it will announce salvation.[2]

Another *Kairos* moment

The challenges that faced the *Kairos* theologians have much in common with the challenges raised, for churches, by the encounter with HIV and AIDS. For many of us, this encounter has proved to be a similar "*Kairos* moment," exposing the fault-lines in our various societies and institutions and challenging existing theological, ethical, and ecclesiological certainties. *The Kairos Document* came down firmly on the side of Prophetic Theology: but the fact remains that there were human rights abuses on all three sides, and Christians were involved in them. As Sally Smith implies, in Chapter 2, our churches are part of the solution, but they can also be part of the problem. We are left with the challenge of dealing with this paradoxical situation.

For HIV and AIDS, too, present us with a *Kairos* moment. Thirty years into the epidemic, with "carnage among young women,"[3] and up to half of all young adults (in some places) infected with HIV, the "signs of the times" would point to a "crisis" in the real sense, meaning a time of fear and emergency, but also a moment of opportunity. This is a time to face realities, a time to stop hiding from the truths exposed by the epidemic, and from the kinds of attitudes and abuses that result in the stigmatization and victimization of those who are well known, now, to be particularly vulnerable to it. One after another, the writers of these essays have sought answers to such difficult questions. What opportunities are we neglecting when we judge those who are most at risk to be beyond the pale, not just of human compassion and mercy but also of careful and targeted public health measures? How do we avoid cheapening the language of rights by allowing it to become a tool for individualism, or for prioritizing the "rights" of one group in ways that deny the broader requirements of social justice?

Saying "yes" to grace

Turning to the gospels, we find Jesus facing similar challenges. The scriptures show his ministry to be one of inclusion, tolerance, and mercy. He attacked the cynicism of authorities who attempted to defend unjust structures, and condemned the legalism of those who put the letter of the law before the requirement to protect the poor and vulnerable. He showed compassion for those who sinned, and exposed the hypocrisy of those who sought to ostracize or demonize them. Again and again, he made people "see" things differently, for example accusing hearers of obsessing about the splinter in another person's eye while ignoring the plank that blocked their own vision (Matt. 7:3-5). Repeatedly, we find him exposing uncomfortable truths in ways that send the authorities away so angry that they want to kill him.

Relating Jesus' ministry to our own contexts, contextual theologian Stephen Bevans suggests that two basic theological orientations or perspectives are available. One of them focuses on failure and sin, setting unrealistic standards of behaviour and then condemning those who fall short of achieving them.[4] In this view, culture and human experience need either radical transformation or total replacement. Grace cannot build on or replace nature, because human nature is basically corrupt. Bevans contrasts this with the orientation that sees the world as a grace-filled reality through which God reveals God's self. In this view, culture and human experience are generally good, allowing grace to build on nature because it is in the experience of grace that human nature becomes free and therefore authentically human.

It is this view we would seek to promote in this publication. It does not mean that we have to suspend our capacity for discerning good from bad. What it does mean is that God's love is total and inclusive; that God's forgiveness is limitless; and that everyone, by virtue of being human, has an inalienable right to be treated with dignity. Accordingly, at this *kairos* moment, let us reflect on the words of Rev. 3:22: "Let anyone who has an ear listen to what the Spirit is saying to the churches."

Notes

Prologue

1. Pope Francis, *Evangelii Gaudium: Apostolic Exhortation to the Bishops, Clergy, Consecrated Persons and the Lay Faithful on the Proclamation of the Gospel in Today's World*, 24 November 2013 (Vatican Press), #190, at: http://w2.vatican.va/content/dam/francesco/pdf/apost_exhortations/documents/papa-francesco_esortazione-ap_20131124_evangelii-gaudium_en.pdf.

Chapter 2: Part of the Solution and Part of the Problem?

1. This is a personal reflection on Sally Smith's role as UNAIDS advisor on partnership with faith-based organizations. More technical information on HIV and human rights can be found in the references, recommended reading, and resources sections of this book.

2. A. Tomkins et al., "Controversies in Faith and Health Care," *The Lancet*, 7 July 2015, at: http://www.thelancet.com/journals/lancet/article/PIIS0140-6736(15)60252-5/abstract.

3. Rowan Williams, "Human Rights and Religious Faith," paper presented at the World Council of Churches, Geneva, 28 February 2012, at: http://rowanwilliams.archbishopofcanterbury.org/articles.php/2370/human-rights-and-religious-faith#sthash.eJLvUqkF.dpuf.

4. Michel Sidibé, "Coalition of the Daring: Coming Together for a New Strategy of Sustainability," Executive Director's report at the opening of the 36th meeting of the UNAIDS Programme Coordinating Board, 30 June 2015, Geneva: at: http://www.unaids.org/sites/default/files/media_asset/20150630_EXDreport_PCB36_en.pdf.

5. We Will Speak Out Coalition, at: http://www.wewillspeakout.org/.

6. Treatment access for children has lagged behind adults, however, even though the situation has improved in recent years. The proportion of children living with HIV who receive antiretroviral therapy more than doubled between 2010 and 2014 (from 14% to 32%), but coverage remains notably lower than it does for adults (41%). As a result of these improvements, new HIV infections among children have been reduced by 58% since 2000. Although 520,000 new infections occurred among children in 2000, the figure plummeted to 220 000 in 2014. See: "How AIDS Changed Everything," UNAIDS (2015), at: http://www.unaids.org/sites/default/files/media_asset/MDG6Report_en.pdf.

7. Cheryl Overs, "Empowerment, Citizenship and Redemption? Economic Programmes and Policies for Female Sex Workers," *Participation, Power and Social Change* (blog), 28 October 2014, at: https://participation-power.wordpress.com/2014/10/28/empowerment-citizenship-and-redemption-economic-programmes-and-policies-for-female-sex-workers/.

8. "Together We Must Do More: My Personal Commitment to Action," *Religious Leadership in Response to HIV*, at: http://www.hivcommitment.net/.

9. Michel Sidibé, "Churches: Barricades against Exclusion," WCC 10th Assembly (31 October 2013), Busan, Republic of Korea, at: http://www.oikoumene.org/en/resources/documents/assembly/2013-busan/plenary-presentations/speech-by-michel-sidibe-executive-director-of-unaids.

10. Luiz Loures, UNAIDS-Caritas Internationalis Joint Consultation with Catholic Church-related and Other FBOs on Expansion of Anti-Retroviral Treatment, 25 February 2014, Rome, Italy, available at: http://hiv.jliflc.com/resources/unaids-caritas-internationalis-joint-consultation-catholic-church-related-fbos-expansion-anti-retroviral-treatment/.

11. UNAIDS, *A Call to Action Faith for Sexual and Reproductive Health and Reproductive Rights Post 2015 Development Agenda*, 19 September 2014, at: http://www.unfpa.org/sites/default/files/resource-pdf/Faith%20leaders%27%20call%20to%20action.pdf.

Chapter 3: Why Stigma Matters

1. The People Living with HIV Stigma Index, at: http://www.stigmaindex.org/
2. See www.frameworkfordialogue.net.

Chapter 5: Health Care, HIV, and Human Rights

1. "Faith-based health-care," *The Lancet*, 7 July 2015, at: http://www.thelancet.com/series/faith-based-health-care.

2. "10 Reasons Why Human Rights Should Occupy the Centre of the Global AIDS Struggle,"at: http://www.hivhumanrightsnow.org/10-reasons/ and http://www.hivhumanrightsnow.org/10-reasons/rhetoric-vs-real-action/.

3. "The Protection of Human Rights Is the Way to Protect the Public's Health," at: http://www.hivhumanrightsnow.org/10-reasons/public-health/.

4. Transgender People and HIV (World Health Organization Policy Brief, July 2015). http://www.who.int/hiv/pub/transgender/transgender-hiv-policy/en/

5. "The Evidence for Addressing Key Populations," Key Populations Action Plan (2014–2017), Global Fund to Fight AIDS, Tuberculosis, and Malaria. http://www.theglobalfund.org/documents/publications/other/Publication_KeyPopulations_ActionPlan_en.

6. *Stories of Stigma, Stories of Hope: Experiences of Pregnant Women and Mothers Living with HIV* (ICASO, 2013). http://www.icaso.org/?file=23935.

7. *The Ecumenical Response to HIV/AIDS in Africa: Plan of Action* (Geneva, WCC, 2001). http://www.wcc-coe.org/wcc/news/press/01/hiv-aids-plan.html

8. *Mukono – Kampala Declaration*, EHAIA, 2001-2003 Statements from Church Leaders' Consultation (WCC), at: http://www.wcc-coe.org/wcc/what/mission/ehaia-html/uganda-mukono-kampala-declaration-e.html.

9. Ibid.

10. "AIDS and the Churches," WCC Excutive Committee, Reyjavik Iceland, 15-19 September 1986, available at http://www.oikoumene.org/en/resources/documents/wcc-programmes/justice-diakonia-and-responsibility-for-creation/ehaia/world-council-of-churches-statements-and-studies/executive-committee-statement.

11. *Together We Must Still Do More: Second Round of Reporting on the Fulfillment of the Personal Commitment to Action on HIV,* Ecumenical Advocacy Alliance (December 2013).

12. "Make Your Personal Commitment to Action," Ecumenical Advocacy Alliance, at: http://www.e-alliance.ch/index833a.html?id=430

13. A discussion with Rev. Canon Gideon Byamugisha, Founder, African Network of Religious Leaders Living with or Personally Affected by HIV/AIDS, 2003.

14. Archbishop Desmond Tutu, "Made for Goodness." *The Huffington Post,*12 January 2012, at: http://www.huffingtonpost.com/desmond-tutu/made-for-goodness_b_1199864.html.

Chapter 6: Reflecting on the Role of Networks of People Living with HIV

1. This reflection is based on a phone interview with Callie Long.

Chapter 10: From Apartheid Activism to AIDS Advocacy

1. This article is written by Callie Long based on an interview with J. Cochrane, 23 September 2014.

2. The United Democratic Front (UDF), formed in 1983, was one of the most important anti-apartheid organizations in the 1980s, and comprised several hundred churches, civic, students', workers', and other national, regional and local organizations. It has boasted some three million members who united under its banner of "UDF Unites, Apartheid Divides."

3. C. Villa-Vicencio and M. Soko, *Conversations in Transition: Leading South African Voices* (Cape Town: David Philip, 2012).

Chapter 11: "Let Grace Be Total"

1. "Let Grace Be Total" (LGBT), UCCP Statement on Lesbian, Gay, Bisexual, Transgender (LGBT) Concerns, 27 May 2014, available at http://www.peaceucc.org/let-grace-be-total-the-ucc-philippiness-initial-statement-on-lgbt-concerns/.

Chapter 12: Stigma, HIV, and Diverse Sexuality

1. "Syndemic" may be defined as a set of linked health problems involving two or more afflictions, interacting synergistically, and contributing to excess burden of disease in a population. Syndemics occur when health-related problems cluster by person, place, or time.

2. "Affirm Diversity: Defend the Rights of Sexual Minorities: A Call for Indian Faith Communities," National Council of Churches in India, 2 June 2014, at: http://www.nccindia.in/index.php/ncci-news/archive/394-affirm-diversity-defend-the-rights-of-sexual-minorities-a-call-for-indian-faith-communities.html.

3. "Uppsala Abrahamic Faith Statement on Human Dignity and Human Sexuality," Interfaith Dialogue on Human Dignity and Human Sexuality (3–8 February 2015), *Svenska Kyrkan*, at: https://www.svenskakyrkan.se/uppsala-festival-of-theology

Chapter 14: As Science Advances . . . the Human Heart Hardens

1. This article has been translated from Portuguese.

2. Como vamos derrotar a Aids? http://revistagalileu.globo.com/Revista/
noticia/2015/10/como-vamos-derrotar-aids.html

Chapter 16: Living by Faith in Challenging Times

1. This contribution is a shortened version of a sermon given by Fr Garth
Minott. It was inspired by readings taken from Chapters 1 and 2 of the Book
of Wisdom.

2. Stephen Pattison, *A Critique of Pastoral Care* (London: SCM Press
Ltd., 1988), 103.

3. John Wilkinson, *Christian Ethics in Health Care* (Edinburgh: The
Handsel Press, 1988).

Chapter 17: The Redemption of God's Good Gift of Sexuality

1. Kapya Kaoma, *The US Christian Right and the Attack on Gays in Africa*,
at: http://www.huffingtonpost.com/rev-kapya-kaoma/the-us-christian-right-
an_b_387642.html.

2. Interview with Desmond Tutu, 2000, at: http://www.indcatholicnews.
com/news.php?viewStory=8134

3. See Marlena Graves, "It's not a Matter of Obeying the Bible":
Eight Questions for Walter Brueggemann," On *Faith*, 9 Jan. 2015, at:
http://www.faithstreet.com/onfaith/2015/01/09/walter-brueggemann-
church-gospel-bible/35739.

Chapter 18: The Image of God

1. Individual quotations in this essay are direct quotations from participants in the EAA colloquium. In one case, the speaker's name has been
changed to protect their identity.

2. Colin Gunton, *The One, the Three and the Many* (Cambridge University Press, 1993), 3.

Chapter 19: Gender Inequality and Human Rights

1. Daniela Gennrich et al., Pietermaritzburg Agency for Christian
Social Action (PACSA) Research Report: *Churches and HIV/AIDS* (Pietermaritzburg: PACSA, 2004). http://micahnetwork.org/library/hiv-aids/
pacsa-research-project-churches-and-hivaids

2. Kwazulu-Natal Church AIDS Network (KZNCAN), *Churches and HIV/AIDS: A Research on KwaZulu-Natal Christian Council* (KZNCC), unpublished report, 2009.

3. Jonathan M. Mann, *Human Rights and AIDS: The Future of the pandemic*, 30 J. Marshall L. Rev. 195 (1996), at http://repository.jmls.edu/cgi/viewcontent.cgi?article=1659&context=lawreview.

4. Stephen B. Bevans, *Models of Contextual Theology*. P. 1-2 Maryknoll: Orbis Books 1992: 1-2.

5. Women and AIDS: An extract from the AIDS epidemic update December 2004, at: http://data.unaids.org/gcwa/jc986-epiextract_en.pdf.

6. Musimbi R.A. Kanyoro, *Introducing Feminist Cultural Hermeneutics: An African Perspective* (London: Sheffield Academic Press, 2002), 18.

7. Also described by Bujo, "The human being does not become human by *cogito* (thinking) but by *relatio* (relationship) and *cognatio* (kinship) The fundamental principle of this ethics is not *cogito ergo sum* (I think, so I am), but rather cognatus sum ergo sum (I am related, so I am). B. Bujo, *The Ethical Dimension of Community: The African Model and the Dialogue between North and South* (Nairobi: Pauline Publications Africa, 1998), 54.

8. WHO, "Why Gender and Health?" at: http://apps.who.int/gender/genderandhealth/en/index.html.

9. Leonardo Boff, *Trinity and Society* (Oregon: Wipf & Stock Publishers, 1998).

Epilogue

1. *Kairos* theologians, *The Kairos Document: Challenge to the Church*, 2nd ed. (London, Catholic Institute for International Relations, 1986), 55, at http://ujamaa.ukzn.ac.za/Libraries/manuals/The_Kairos_Documents.sflb.ashx.

2. Ibid., 63-64.

3. Stephen Lewis, formerly UN Special Envoy for HIV and AIDS in Africa.

4. Stephen B. Bevans, *Models of Contextual Theology* (Maryknoll: Orbis, 2002), 16.

Resources

The aim of this publication is to open up an issue many people find difficult and to introduce readers to individuals who are struggling to make sense of it. In doing this, a primary aim was to point readers to many relevant resources that are available. For a start, each of our writers has included references to important sources on which they personally have drawn. Some of them have also included short lists of works they belive to be of particular importance. In this section, we are seeking to provide pointers to further material you may find interesting or useful. Section 1 is a list of some of the basic international documents and protocols – mainly United Nations – that provide the building blocks of our understanding of human rights in our time. Section 2 contains a short list of general commentaries on human rights theory and practice. Section 3 consists of a long list of sources and materials, proposed by our writers, in which the issue of HIV and religion is generally addressed. In Section 4, we have tried to provide links to some, at least, of the wealth of training and educational material that is available, much of it developed by our partner organizations in producing this book, and nowadays widely available online. And because religion and human rights have enjoyed a longstanding (if not always harmonious) relationship, Section 5 makes some suggestions about where readers might go in search of further understanding.

In this rapidly expanding field of knowledge, it would be impossible to include all relevant publications. Our aim has been to supplement what we are offering in this publication and to guide you to the sources you are likely to need in your own life and work. We have needed to choose. So rather than omit the very many resources people have suggested, we are inviting interested readers to access further material via the weblink www.oikoumene.org/dignity-freedom-grace.

1. Core Documents on Human Rights and the Law

The Core International Human Rights Instruments and Their Monitoring Bodies. United Nation Human Rights. http://www.cesr.org/article. php?id=271.

Declaration of Commitment on HIV/AIDS Adopted by the General Assembly. UN News Center, 2001. www.un.org/ga/aids/coverage/FinalDeclarationHIVAIDS.html.

HIV and the Law: Risks, Rights and Health. UNDP, 2012 http://www. undp.org/content/undp/en/home/librarypage/hiv-aids/hiv-and-the-law--risks--rights---health.html.

Human Rights and the Law. UNAIDS, 2014. http://www.unaids.org/sites/default/files/media_asset/2014unaids guidancenote_humanrightsandthelaw_en.pdf

Human Rights Documents. United Nation Human Rights. http:// ap.ohchr.org/documents/dpage_e.aspx?m=106.

International Covenant on Civil and Political Rights. United Nation Human Rights. http://www.ohchr.org/EN/ProfessionalInterest/Pages/CCPR. aspx.

International Covenant on Economic, Social and Cultural Rights. United Nations Human Rights. http://www.ohchr.org/EN/ProfessionalInterest/Pages/CESCR.aspx.

The International Bill of Human Rights: A Brief History of the International Covenants on Human Rights (and Optional Protocol). New York, N.Y.: United Nations Office of Public Information, 1977.

Political Declaration on HIV and AIDS: Intensifying our Efforts to Eliminate HIV and AIDS. Resolution of the United Nations General Assembly, adopted 8 July 2011. http://www.unaids.org/sites/default/files/sub_landing/files/20110610_UN_A-RES-65-277_en.pdf

Reduction of HIV-Related Stigma and Discrimination. UNAIDS, 2014.

Ten Reasons Why Human Rights Should Occupy the Centre of the Global AIDS Struggle. In *Human Rights and HIV/AIDS: Now More Than Ever.* http://www.hivhumanrightsnow.org/10-reasons/.

The Universal Declaration of Human Rights. UN. http://www.un.org/en/documents/udhr/.

Universal Human Rights Instruments by Category. Women with Disabilities Australia. http://wwda.org.au/issues/unhrt/hrins1/.

See UNAIDS web page for a series of additional materials on HIV and the Law: http://www.unaids.org/en/ourwork/programme-branch/rightsgenderpreventioncommunitymobilizationdepartment/humanrightsdivision

2. Selected Background Literature on Human Rights

Clapham, Andrew. *Human Rights: A Very Short Introduction.* Oxford: Oxford University Press, 2007

Drinan, Robert F. *The Mobilization of Shame: A World View of Human Rights.* New Haven: Yale University Press, 2001.

Holder, Cindy. *Human Rights: The Hard Questions.* Cambridge University Press, 2013.

Mahoney, John. *The Challenge of Human Rights: Origin, Development, and Significance.* Malden, Mass.: Blackwell Pub., 2007.

Mahoney, Kathleen E., and Paul Mahoney (eds). *Human Rights in the Twenty-first Century: A Global Challenge.* Dordrecth; Boston: M. Nijhoff, 1993.

Nussbaum, Martha C. *Hiding from Humanity: Disgust, Shame and the Law.* Princeton N.J.: Princeton University Press. 2004.

3. Resources on HIV and Religion

Bartelink, Brenda, and Erik Meinema. *A Mapping on Sexuality, Human Rights and the Role of Religious Leaders: Exploring the Potential for Dialogue.* HIVOS, Knowledge Centre Religion and Development, 2015.

Byamugisha, Gideon B., John Joshva Raj, and Ezra Chitando (eds). *Is the Body of Christ HIV Positive? New Ecclesiological Christologies in the Context of HIV Positive Communities.* Indian Society for Promoting Christian Knowledge, 2014.

Chitando, Ezra (ed.) *Abundant Life: The Churches and Sexuality* (EHAIA series.) Geneva: WCC Publications, 2015.

Clifford, Paula. *Theology and the HIV/AIDS Epidemic.* London: Christian Aid, 2004.

Cochranc, James R., et al. (eds). *When Religion and Health Align: Mobilising Religious Health Assets for Transformation.* Pietermaritzburg: Cluster Publications, 2011.

Dube, Musa W. (ed). *HIV/AIDS and the Curriculum: Methods of Integrating HIV/AIDS in Theological Programmes.* Geneva: WCC Publications, 2003.

Haddad, Beverley (ed). *Religion and HIV and AIDS: Charting the Terrain.* Pietermaritzburg: University of KwaZulu Natal Press, 2011.

Kanyoro, Musimbi. *Grant Me Justice! HIV/AIDS and Gender Readings of the Bible.* Edited by Musa W. Dube. Pietermaritzburg: Cluster Publications, 2004.

Fuller, Jon D., and James F. Keenan. "The Language of Human Rights and Social Justice in the Face of HIV-AIDS." *Budhi: A Journal of Ideas and Culture* 8:1-2 (2004). http://journals.ateneo.edu/ojs/budhi/article/view/670/667.

Gill, Robin (ed). *Reflecting Theologically on AIDS: A Global Challenge.* Londen: SCM Press, 2007.

Gravgaard, Elsebeth, and Martin Rosenkilde. *A Vicious Circle of Vulnerability: Orphans, Vulnerable Children and Youth in Relation to HIV and AIDS.* Copenhagen: DanChurchAid, N.D.

Luginaah, Isaac N., Emmanuel K. Yiridoe, and Mary-Margaret Taabazuing. "From Mandatory to Voluntary Testing: Balancing Human Rights, Religious and Cultural Values, and HIV/AIDS Prevention in Ghana." *Social Science and Medicine* 61:8 (2005), 1689–1700.

Manning, Greg. "Coverage for All Who Are Marginalized." *The Ecumenical Review* 63:4 (2011), 443–55. DOI: 10.1111/j.1758-6623.2011.00136.x.

Monshipouri, Mahmood, and Travis Trapp. "HIV/AIDS, Religion, and Human Rights: A Comparative Analysis of Bangladesh, Indonesia, and Iran." *Human Rights Review* 13:2 (2012), 187–204.

Okyere-Manu, Beatrice. "HIV and AIDS as a Human Rights Challenge to Faith Communities in Pietermaritzburg, South Africa." In *Religion and Human Rights Global Challenges from Intercultural Perspectives*, ed. Wilhelm Gräb and Lars Charbonnier, 187-200. Berlin/Boston: Walter De Gruyter, 2015.

Paiva, V., J. Garcia, L.F. Rios, A.O. Santos, V. Terto, and M. Munõz-Laboy. "Religious Communities and HIV Prevention: An Intervention Study Using a Human Rights-based Approach." *Global Public Health* 5:3 (2010), 280–94.

Paterson, Gillian (ed). *HIV Prevention: A Global Theological Conversation.* Geneva: EAA, 2009.

4. Resources Suitable for Groups

In addition to the material introduced below, we recommend that you make use of the group-questions that appear at the end of the chapters in this book.

CAFOD (Catholic Fund for Overseas Development)
CAFOD's toolkit of Selected Resources for Faith Leaders Responding to HIV-related Stigma and Discrimination, Africa, Asia and Latin America is listed here: http://www.cafod.org.uk/content/download/14673/116660/version/1/file/HIV-Resources-FaithLeaders-AfricaAsiaLatinAm.pdf.

Ecumenical Advocacy Alliance
The following EAA publications can be accessed on this link:
   http://www.e-alliance.ch/en/s/resources/eaa-publications/index.html,
   DVD on Religious Leadership
   My Personal Commitment to Action
   HIV Prevention: A Global Theological Conversation
   Exploring Solutions: How to Talk about HIV Prevention in the Church
   AIDS Related Stigma: Thinking Outside the Box - The Theological Challenge

EHAIA (the WCC's Ecumenical HIV and AIDS Initiatives and Advocacy)
   EHAIA has many useful resources, which may be found on this link: http://www.oikoumene.org/en/what-we-do/ehaia/documents

The Lancet
The Lancet's series on Faith-based health-care can be accessed on this link:
   http://www.thelancet.com/series/faith-based-health-care. *The Lancet*, July 7, 2015

Strategies for Hope
You will find the Strategies for Hope "Called to Care" tool-kit of resources listed on this link: http://www.stratshope.org/resources/called_to_care
   These include:
   Open Secret: People Facing Up to HIV and AIDS in Uganda (2000);
   Journeys of Faith: Church-based Responses to HIV and AIDS in Three Southern African Countries (2002);
   Positive Voices: Religious Leaders Living with or Personally Affected by HIV and AIDS (2005).

UNICEF
UNICEF, What Religious Leaders Can Do about AIDS. At: http://www.uni-cef.org/media/files/Religious_leaders_Aids.pdf

United Church of Christ (UCC) with Unitarian Universalist Association
Our Whole Lives is a faith-based, life-span, age-appropriate, comprehensive sexuality education curriculum. It may be accessed via this link: www.ucc.org/owl

5. Religion and Human Rights Literature

An-Na'im, Abdullahi A., Jerald D. Gort, Henry Jansen, and Hendrik M. Vroom (eds). *Human Rights and Religious Values: An Uneasy Relationship?* Amsterdam: Editions Rodopi, 1995.

Bloom, Irene, J. Paul Martin, and Wayne L. Proudfoot (eds). *Religious Diversity and Human Rights.* New York: Columbia University Press, 1996.

Botta, Alejandro F. *The Bible and the Hermeneutics of Liberation.* Atlanta: Society of Biblical Literature, 2009.

Bucar, Elizabeth M., and Barbara Barnett (eds). *Does Human Rights Need God?* Grand Rapids, Mich.: William B. Eerdmans Pub., 2005.

Chitando, Ezra, and Sophia Chirongoma (eds). *Justice Not Silence. Churches Facing Sexual And Gender-Based Violence.* Stellenbosch: Sun Press, 2013.

Cronin, Kieran. *Rights and Christian Ethics.* Cambridge: Cambridge University Press, 2009.

Donahue, James, and M. Theresa Moser (eds). *Religion, Ethics and the Common Good.* 41st ed. Mystic, Conn.: Twenty-third Publications, 1996.

Gaay Fortman, B. de."Religion and Human Rights: Mutually Exclusive or Supportive?" *Studies in Interreligious Dialogue* 6:1 (1996), 98–110.

Getz, Lorine M., *Human Rights and the Global Mission of the Church.* Cambridge, Mass.: Boston Theological Institute, 1985.

Ghanea, Nazila, Alan Stephens, and Raphael Walden (eds). *Does God Believe in Human Rights? Essays on Religion and Human Rights.* Volume 5 of Studies in *Religion, Secular Beliefs and Human Rights.* Leiden: Martinus Nijhoff Publishers, 2007.

Gustafson, Carrie, and Peter H. Juviler (eds). *Religion and Human Rights: Competing Claims?* Armonk, N.Y.: M.E. Sharpe, 1999.

Haas, Peter J., William H. Brackney, Muddathir 'Abd Al-Rahim, Harold Coward, and Robert E. Florida' (eds). *Human Rights and the World's Major Religions*. Westport, Conn.: Praeger, 2005.

Haughey, J. C. "Responsibility for Human Rights: Contributions from Bernard Lonergan." *Theological Studies* 63 (2002), 764–85. doi: 10.1177/004056390206300405

Hennelly, Alfred T., ed. *Human Rights in the Americas: The Struggle for Consensus*. Washington, D.C.: Georgetown University Press, 1982.

Hollenbach, David. *Claims in Conflict: Retrieving and Renewing the Catholic Human Rights Tradition*. New York: Paulist Press, 1979.Holman, Susan R. *Beholden: Religion, Global Health, and Human Rights*. Oxford University Press. 2015.

Ilesanmi, Simeon O. "Human Rights Discourse in Modern Africa: A Comparative Religious Ethical Perspective." *The Journal of Religious Ethics* 23:2 (1995), 293–322.

Karam, Azza. "On Faith, Health and Tensions An Overview from an Inter-Governmental Perspective." *The Heythrop Journal* 55:6 (2014), 1069–1079. doi: 10.1111/heyj.12217

Kitanović, Mag. Elizabeta (ed). *European Churches Engaging in Human Rights: Present Challenges and Training Material*. Brussels: Church and Society Commission of CEC, 2012.

Kung, Hans, and Jurgen Moltmann (eds). *The Ethics of World Religions and Human Rights*. 2nd ed. London: SCM Press, 1990.

MacArthur, Kathleen Walker. *The Bible and Human Rights*. Rev. ed. New York: Woman's Press, 1949.

Reed, Esther. "Human Rights, the Churches and the Common Good." *Political Theology* 3:1 (2001), 9-21. doi: 10.1558/poth.v3i1.9

Regan, Ethna. *Theology and the Boundary Discourse of Human Rights*. Washington, DC: Georgetown University Press, 2010.

Reuver, Marc (ed). *Human Rights: A Challenge to Theology*. Rome: CCIA & IDOC International, 1983.

Rouner, Leroy S. *Human Rights and the World's Religions*. Notre Dame, Ind.: University of Notre Dame Press, 1988.

Ruland, Vernon. *Conscience across Borders: An Ethics of Global Rights and Religious Pluralism*. San Francisco, Cal.: University of San Francisco/Association of Jesuit University Presses, 2002.